EMS

EARN MONEY SLEEPING

SEMON STROBOS

Copyright © 2009 Semon Strobos

All rights reserved.

ISBN: 978-1499360097

OLD MEDIC JOKE ABOUT 24 HOUR SHIFTS:
"YOU KNOW WHAT EMS STANDS FOR?"
"EMERGENCY MEDICAL……SOMETHING?"
"NO: EARN MONEY SLEEPING

CONTENTS

1

The first full arrest I ran—full cardiac arrest—was at 2 AM in the morning, after 18 hours of running calls. We were "getting hammered," as EMTs call it. We work 24/48: 24 hours on, 48 off, seven days a week, 365 days a year, excluding our two week vacation. Among many superstitions—anything serious that can't be controlled breeds superstitions—medics believe they are either white clouds or shit magnets. When my new partner, Trish, the EMT Basic who assists me (the paramedic), asked me which I was, I didn't know what to say. I didn't endorse the superstition, but in all honesty I hadn't been visited with many ugly calls, which is why I took the busier post where she worked. Sitting around waiting for something awful to happen isn't nearly as much fun as immersion. Waiting is scarier.

"White sheep, I guess," I'd allowed.

Trish was pleased. The longer your tenure, the less shit you're in the mood for. Though the big ones still get your attention.

So when the tones went off for the 10th time, she awoke and said, "White sheep, my ass. You're fired." Trish used to be a long haul trucker so she drives like a bat on PCP. I had to ask her to slow down, owing to being in fear of my life, screaming a two lane country road "riding the governor" which caps the rig at 92 mph so it won't burn out its engine.

The tones, and the radio "traffic" in general, I consider to be among the most romantic aspects of an obviously romantic profession. We live with the radio. It's never out of earshot. Awake or asleep, a medic hears his unit number called. The radio tells all of us, all on the same channel, where to go, what to expect, and we use it to call for rescue, get information, let Dispatch know where we are and what we're doing at all times. We call "in route," "on scene," "transporting," "destination" and "clear" on every call. It sends us out on calls or posts us to other locations, asks us our status, admonishes us to call in patient information. We ask it which hospitals are open, what the sheriff's officers' ETA is (even though they never say), ask for directions when it gets us lost.

When I was a kid there was a TV show called Highway Patrol which featured Broderick Crawford, a character actor who looked like a bulldog with a bad hangover. He was forever leaning with noir glamour on his "unit' calling "ten codes" into his radio, usually "ten four." 40 years later things haven't changed a whit, and years after 9/11 we still can't talk to law enforcement. Homeland Security never issued new radio channels. At that time, age 10, I had no desire to be a fireman or policeman, but I used to be more mature.

The emergency call goes like this. "WeeOweeOweeO....Medic 203 prepare to copy emergency traffic, map grid 714 Fox 3, 714 Fox 3" referring to the square on our map.

We press our button and say "203" or "Go ahead."

"Medic 203, respond code 3 (lights and sirens, no matter what the chief complaint is: 'you call, we haul') to 2214 Smith Road, 2214 Smith Road, map grid 714 Fox 3, 714 Fox 3, for a 36 year old female, cardiac arrest. CPR in progress."

"Copy. ETA ten or less."

For a full arrest a backup unit is dispatched unless we cancel it, saying we have a three man crew (a student on board) or a first responder who can help. Transporting a full arrest requires at least three trained responders. So two flaming units cry and moan through the night racing different roads in the sleeping dark. (Siren tones are named "wail," "yelp" and "chatter.") In the long dark night of the soul it's always three o'clock in the morning. From dark wine and a thousand roses runs the hour rushing into the dream of night. And Scott Fitzgerald and Rilke were merely describing insomnia and love, not life and death.

We pulled up at a rundown little house on a dirt back road behind a flashing fire truck. I would've been icy with fear even if Trish had not been flying at ground level.

Wrenched out of uneasy sleep to fight death. Hoping to remember my algorithms, perform my interventions successfully and not make any horrible mistakes. Do no harm. Only my second intubation of a human patient. The first with no backer.

We've beaten the volunteer fireman first responders this time. I hop out, haul the cardiac monitor from the side door and trot in behind a fireman. On the filthy carpet in the living room a dark haired slight woman lies on her back straddled by a police officer doing chest compressions. I get the fireman to take over while squeezing the paddles to her chest, left midaxillary, and right under the collarbone. She does not show a shockable rhythm. She's in asystole, a flat line indicating no electrical activity in her heart at all. The chances of bringing back a person found down in asystole are close to nil. Bringing her back with reasonably intact brain function is even less likely. 36 years old, no medical conditions, found by her husband within a half hour or less of last seen alive. Still, I do not see dependent lividity, the red or magenta or blue stains indicating blood has pooled and coagulated, and can no longer be circulated, so I follow the indicated algorithm, asystole.

By this time Trish has brought in the airway bag, pulled out the adult bag valve mask (BVM), put it together, attached it to oxygen and is supervising a fireman holding it to the patient's nose and mouth, head tipped appropriately, and ventilating at 10 breaths a minute. Nowadays we do 5. Algorithms change. The other fireman is still compressing her chest at a rate of 100 times a minute, compressing a third to half down, deep and even pumps. We check the carotid for a good CPR pulse. After five minutes he will tire and need relief. A bodybuilder by the looks, he could go on longer, but not well. For the time being, the least trained caregiver is doing the most important job.

With my partner's help, I pull out the intubation kit, select the middle sized curved blade, Mac 3. I slide the blade under the patient's tongue with my left hand, lift, look for the vocal cords, slide in the endotracheal tube, stiffened by a wire stylette inserted by Trish, using my other hand. Then I pull out the stylette, hold the ET tube in place while she attaches the BVM. She ventilates and I listen over the lungs and stomach to make sure the tube is in the trachea and not the esophagus, watch for chest rise and fall, misting in the tube. Then we tie it down.

You can arrive at the hospital with a mangled patient, you can perpetrate spectacular fuckups and keep your job and license to practice, but arrive with a tube in the wrong hole, you're looking for another livelihood. Almost as bad, the patient will be dead. And horribly bloated. Probably drenched in vomit.

At this point, the backup crew arrived, bringing with them hot steamy diesel air, dead leaves and, as it transpired, a nasty chaos. The other paramedic was a pompous melodramatic bald shaven dude, who, unfortunately, outranked me. He was a Field Training Officer, me just out of the plastic wrap. By protocol this was my call, as first paramedic on scene, but he could take it over if he felt I was making a mess.

It's very difficult for a paramedic not to take over anything he possibly can. Marriages, whatever. Works quite well at emergency scenes and fairly miserably almost everywhere else.

Normal life comes to seem slow, boring, inconsequential. Your mind is back on shift. People are taking too long to make decisions. They're dithering, vain, unfocussed, probably incompetent. Adrenalin and interventions required.

I've moved to the patient's AC, the inner elbow, looking for a vein to cannulate. Jack, the other paramedic, is ordering drugs out, making a huge racket. His plan, which I overhear, is to shoot an ml of 1 to 1000 epinephrine down the ET tube. I know from my paramedic studies—I did very well on the national registry test—that this dosage can be used in infants under some circumstances, but the ET tube should take 2 or 3 ml of 1 to 10.000 epi. Fortunately I have by now got an IV started so we run it wide open and shoot 1 ml of 1 to 10.000 into my catheter instead, so the issue doesn't arise. The ET tube is no longer used at all for meds, now that access is assured with intraosseus needles drilled into bone, but in those days we would try double doses in the ET tube if we couldn't get a vein.

CPR is continuous. We put in 4 rounds of epi at five minute intervals. We alternate with two rounds of atropine for slow heart rates (0). We put in an amp of sodium bicarbonate for acidity. We check her blood sugar. Normal, so no dextrose. We check the cardiac rhythm a couple times. Still asystole. The other medic's partner records every intervention, every test.

Trish, softhearted, is in the next room with the husband by now. He's sobbing, distraught and irrational. If there could be anything worse than finding your young, you thought healthy, wife dead on the floor, it's having a gang of firemen storm in and assault her defenseless body with blows and sharp instruments. I pay no attention to anything except my patient and my algorithm.

We pause, having done everything.

"What do you want to do next?" Jack asks. He's been letting me run the call, which has been flawless so far. It was not a difficult arrest. Access to the patient was simple. She was an easy tube, with no vomit in her airway. She was an easy stick, a healthy young woman with good veins. I had all the trained help I could want.

"Well," I said, "another round of epi and we call it."

Trish told me later the firemen and everyone was shocked. Give up on such a young woman? With the husband beside himself?

One half hour of asystole, with every indicated intervention adequately performed, and no cardiac response whatsoever, means the patient is dead. The family can now say goodbye in their own home, without the alarums and excursions of emergency transport, the huge expense, the false hopes, the cold fluorescent hospital.

Jack overruled me. Which meant we had to put a cervical collar on our corpse so that the neck would not flex and dislodge my tube in route. We had to log roll her onto a backboard and tape blocks beside her head. We had to pick the board up and secure it to a stretcher. We had to load the stretcher onto an ambulance. We had to speed lights and sirens to a distant emergency room. We had to pretend we were doing adequate chest compressions during all this movement. We had to call the facility and tell them we were en route with a full arrest, CPR in progress. One medic drove, three in back continued to 1) ventilate the patient with the bag valve mask, 2) hang from the swaying monkey bar with one hand and try to do chest compressions with the other, and 3) keep shooting more epinephrine into my IV. The fact that none of this works very well compared to the relative order of the living room before Jack got there didn't really matter since the patient was unsalvageable by now anyway.

Do do this at home, by the way. No special training required. No excuses. "I didn't know CPR." If you don't particularly care for French kissing dead people, just leave out the part where you tip his head back and breathe two breaths into his mouth, while pinching his nose, after every 30 compressions. Just straddle the body, put the heel of your hand in the middle of his chest with the other hand on top and pump fluidly 100 times a minute, compressing the chest a third to half way. If you're not into the female superior position, you can kneel beside the patient, but it will strain your lower back.

Jack really enjoyed this part. We rolled the stretcher into the ER with him standing on the footrail, pumping chest. After the MD had pronounced—who expected anything else?—Jack put both his hands up in the air. Some kind of benediction, I think.

"Stop!" the doc had said to his staff, thrashing in a feeding frenzy, freezing them dead in full flagrante delecti. "Look at the monitor. Does anyone see any kind of rhythm? (Pause) This patient is DEAD." My sentiments exactly.

I'm probably as compassionate as the next guy, and my bedside manner really isn't that bad, but I can easily imagine and rehearse reproaches about my icy heart. "Woo, that's cold, man." Plenty of people are nicer than I am, more helpful, more tactful, more sympathetic,

I'm motivated by professionalism. I want to do the job not just right but perfectly, and faster than anyone else can do it. 25 full arrests. 6 saves.

When I imagine someone reproaching me for lack of sympathy, my response to this imaginary inquisitor—it's never happened in real life—is, "and how many lives have you saved?"

"Well, how many have you?"

"I don't really know. About one a week for five years, depending on how you define it."

Unfortunately I find a lot of this stuff funny. I spend a lot of time laughing with my partners. Maybe it's what keeps us sane, but I think it's the exhilaration. We like our work. We feel good about it.

I remember the doc who met our truck at Wilford Hall Medical Center when we were running in another full arrest.

"Stop," he said as we were wheeling the stretcher into the door. We stopped. We looked at him. He mounted the side of the stretcher and began pumping chest. "Go," he said.

We did. “I saw them doing this on ER,” he confided. “It looked really cool.”

2 YOU CALL, WE HAUL

Probably 85 % of 911 callers do not need emergency transport to a hospital. They don't have a car, the ankle they sprained or broke during the day is keeping them awake and they don't want to wake up a neighbor or relative, they don't have a doctor, they think ambulance transport will shoot them to the top of the line at the ER, whatever. You call, we haul. They don't call us for lethal chest pain, they do call for flu.

We already have universal health care. Anyone can call 911, get an ambulance ride to the hospital of their choice, and be seen by a physician. It may take all day, with no follow up or preventive care, but that just means more calls and more visits.

So we have our frequent flyers. There was Donny Brook, an alcoholic who lived in a rundown farm house, stranded by suburban sprawl, down the street from a porn mega emporium. Donny was good for a call a month. He had some serious medical problems, as alcoholics do, and was a poor historian, so you never knew what you would get when you got there. You never do anyway. There was always the chance he could be bleeding out from burst varices, vomiting blood into his lungs, or breathing agonally from a cranial bleed--both common in alcoholics--but usually it would be one of his psych problems. Unfortunately, medics tend to want patience with psych calls. Psych calls don't fit the blue collar mindset or the macho image: another life saved. Though we see as many as some psychiatrists. A major part of our practice. When I moved from Basic to Paramedic, one of my few regrets was that my Basic partner now took all the psych calls, which I found pretty interesting, and often challenging. My boast is I can get along with anyone for 15 minutes. After that she was the ER's problem. My technique mostly is stay in front of them, keep some but not intrusive eye contact, and let them talk. Everyone wants to explain, to anyone who will listen, exactly and in detail what's bothering them. Few people and fewer psych patients get the full attention they desire.

Distraction is good too. How many kids do you have? You do not want to feed their delusions, though. Not up to you to diagnose, or document their delusional system. "The little green men want you to be quiet and cooperative" is not a good strategy. Better to admit you don't see them and change the subject.

On occasion, a police officer and five strapping firemen plus three medics will be required to hold someone down while I shoot in a cocktail of Haldol and Versed, preferably into a vein. In five minutes my rabid WWF wrestler turns into a pussycat. Snoring pussycat.

The first time they put Haldol into my pharmacopeia I fell in love. No more tying down struggling loons. No more trying to keep psychotic body builders with 'roid rage from hurting themselves or us. It takes one stronger person to subdue someone. Though not me if I can avoid it. But it takes 4 to 6 fireman and officers to do so without hurting anyone. Damn, I thought, seeing the Haldol take effect, I need to give this to the receiving nurse, my partner, my boss.

Once we had to chase Donny across a plowed field, after his mom reported he was delusional and suicidal. This was not as much fun as it might have looked. On the one hand, we did have some employer-sanctioned sport chasing Donny like a cimarron kid over the furrowed black dirt--actually grey or brown in the sun--cutting off his routes of escape. True, we were exempted for a while from responding to mangled vehicles seeping oil and blood, rectal bleeds with blood pressures in their socks, while we dealt with Donny. On the other hand, it was midsummer in Texas. Even standing motionless under a pecan tree will soak your uniform within minutes. Cutting and roping on foot made even our belts and boots slimy and greasy in short order. With no near prospect of a shower or change. Fortunately Donny had no endurance. Footspeed also unexceptional.

This time, though, Donny's mom answered the door. It's always good when people aren't out on the curb waving at you, hyperventilating, when you have to ring doorbells to get their attention. Unless there's no answer, and the caller may be alone inside. Then you have to contemplate breaking and entering, preferably with a police officer in charge, hoping to find a false alarm, rather than a collapsed aortic aneurism or pulmonary embolism. Though I've never once responded to a medic alert to find an actual patient in distress. Their dog or kid hit the alarm button, they don't know what happened, or they're nowhere to be found.

I do remember arriving as second unit at one dropped call. The caller had been talking to our dispatcher about chest pain when the line went dead. The first medic on scene was just standing there on the porch. A really bad neighborhood, where even the cops went in twos. Where even the birds sing bass. Plus at least 50% of households in Texas feature a fire arm, possibly in the grip of a gang member with outstanding warrants, a paranoid schizophrenic, or a deaf and demented German rancher. The medic said there was supposed to be a dog inside, though where did she hear that? No barking. I found an unlocked window and slid in over a table. I held a chair in front of me for a shield. “Nice doggy,” I said in a high placating voice. “Don't shoot, EMS,” I said in a deep calm voice. “Nice doggy. Don't shoot, EMS. Nice doggy....”

I got to the living room where I found, right by the front door on a ratty couch, a fat middle aged woman, still holding the phone to her ear, stone cold dead and blue. I opened the door, pulled her to the floor onto her back and attached the monitor my partner brought in. Asystole. We checked for dependent lividity, initiated CPR. I opened her mouth, dislodging a set of false teeth, to find a virtual lake of vomit. She had aspirated to death, like so many of our full arrests, like Jimi Hendrix and Janis Joplin. Our portable suction really does not work well enough, but I got as much out as I could, and attempted to intubate around the ventilations provided by the BVM and the compressions. Couldn't get the tube. Too fat, no neck. Ventilation via BVM was adequate, though, so we ran the code on her floor, IV epi, everything, and pronounced after half an hour.

Finally Donny's door opened. His mom looked at us, nonplussed.

"What's up?"

"What?"

"Did you call 911?"

"Nooo." She sounded like she wasn't quite sure. I believed her though.

"Well, did Donny call? Where is he?"

"He's in the back, asleep. I think."

We trooped through the house, kicking aside Burger King bags where necessary. In the back bedroom we found Donny supine, mouth agape, snoring raggedly. An unedifying sight. Color, muscle tone, chest rise normal.

"Donny! Hey, Donny! Wake up, man. Come on, buddy." We shook him reasonably gently.

"Whuh," he allowed.

"No, man, you gotta wake up. Talk to me."

"It was like that when I found it."

"Come on, Donny. Did you call EMS?"

The light of consciousness, such as it was, began to dawn. Donny was not happy to see us. Now, instead of sleeping peacefully, he had a headache and a hangover. The light was too bright. Assholes were asking him stupid questions.

"Donny! Did you call 911?'

Doubt wrinkled his brow. The raveled sleeve of care.

"I believe I did," he said. He realized he had brought this on himself like so much in his jinxed life.

"Well, are you all right? What's the matter? What hurts?"

"Yeah," he said. "I mean, nothing."

"Well, what can we do for you? Why did you call us?"

"Uh, well...I don't remember."

We took a signed refusal. We checked him out thoroughly first too, and it's always a risk—suppose he fortuitously has a heart attack in the next hour or remembers he had a seizure or bloody stool?—but he didn't want to go. Can't force him. That's kidnapping.

He went back to sleep and his mom saw us out.

"Well, if anything happens, call us back. Don't hesitate. You have our number?"

"No, no, I don't think I do. Let me get a pen to write it down.'

"I think you can remember it. It's 911."

Yeah, for 5 years my phone number was 911. Way cooler than a vanity plate.

You can get pissed off by people like Donny. It certainly does say something about our expensive medical care. We could deliver as good or better care for half as much if we could triage it to the people who need it. But if Donny got to you, you'd be pissed off most of the time, otherwise known as burnout. Crews are pretty good humored most of the time. By the time you get to a "bullshit call" in the middle of the night, you're fully awake anyway. We kind of enjoy people like Donny. He's funny. Besides, who really wants to run balls to the wall critical catastrophes on every outing? And how would we practice for them except on patients like Donny?

Donny was no worse than the guy we found pacing around outside his house on the sidewalk in the middle of the afternoon. We pulled up beside him, shut off the siren and rolled down the window.

"What's up?"

"I think I may not be able to sleep tonight."

So he dialed 911, not for insomnia, but for anticipated insomnia.

Or the old guy in a sweltering shack who couldn't get out of his chair. His legs were so swollen and discolored he might have had elephantiasis.

What kind of medical problems do you have? He didn't know. They have a gold plated pharmacopeia on hand—the latest antidepressants, nothing generic—paid for by Medicare or Medicaid, but they don't know what the meds are for, or what their family members' are for. They may or may not take them on schedule or get to the pharmacy for refills.

This guy had a whole bag full, including Lasix, a diuretic. He looked like congestive heart failure.

"Have you been taking your Lasix?

"What?'

"Your water pills? Have you been taking your water pills?"

"Naw, they make me pee all the time."

Since it was hard for him to get up, the last thing he wanted was frequent trips to the bathroom. So now he couldn't get up at all.

"Sir, your heart is too weak to get all the water out of your body. So that means you can have water in your lungs, in your legs, or, if you take your pills, in your toilet. The choice is yours."

He claimed no one had ever told him this. This may be true. Family practice docs who take care of the indigent don't have a lot of time to explain things, and their patients tend not to understand or listen. They forget easily. You can see why a physician wouldn't want to get into an hour discussion, complete with blackboard and anatomical doll, on how fluid circulates in your body, with a slow student who didn't realize there was fluid in his body. But it was clear this gentlemen had not made much effort to be informed. You take your body to a doc like you take your car to a mechanic. You don't listen to the explanation. Boring. Not your job. So I make a point of sitting with my patients and explaining what's happening to them, what the guy with chest pain can expect from the hospital, and why. It's reassuring and patients are grateful. Besides the gratitude, I enjoy explaining things. I'm the village explainer. I miss teaching in some ways. Anyone who will gratify me by actually listening is entitled to a free lecture on the subject of my choice. I have many original or valuable insights in many areas and wide reading to back them up. It's a disappointment to me hardly anyone listens, much less acts on my advice. A person strapped down face up on a stretcher in my ambulance has little choice. What you call a captive audience.

Still and all, though, there are calls that get old. "Assault" means no one is really hurt. "Gunshot wound (GSW)", "stabbing," "possible fracture," "head injury" mean someone is hurt. "Assault" means someone is mad at someone, and wants to use the police for revenge or self defense. The cops know this as well as we do, so they take their time responding. And on psych calls and assaults we have to wait for them to secure the scene before we make it. So, 2 AM, we're staged around the corner from the address, waiting for SO (Sheriff) to show up. Then we get to meet yet another dysfunctional family. At first they're interesting, but, pace Tolstoy, after a while they're all the same. Annoying. You can see why someone might want to punch one or more of them. Then we either get to do an exam, and take a signed refusal, clearing the sheriff's officers of medical liability--why not? they protect us too--or we take someone with a bruised cheek into the ER so she can build a court case against her husband. Which he richly deserves, and which she ought to do, and which we ought to help her with. But not what any sane person feels like doing at three in the morning after two hours sleep. You call we haul.

3 DEATH

"You're the angel of death," the ER nurse said to me admiringly as we crossed paths when I was walking out of Wilford Hall Medical Center ER after bringing her another catastrophe. It had been one after the other the last weeks.

Her tone was only mildly awed, only a little impressed, mostly pleased and friendly. There's nothing a good ER nurse enjoys more than a catastrophe. She has a whole team around her and she likes her job. As for me in the field, not so much. I'm in charge, less well trained, less equipped and with only a Basic partner and a couple firemen to help. Bless their excellent hearts. It's not unlike the way my 6 year old son felt about running a rapid on my lap in our kayak. It had been a lot of fun, looking back from just downstream. The passage itself was really cool too, though scary, as long as everything went well. But the anticipation, not so much. And when things go wrong, even not fatally, even correctably wrong, it's terrifying. It has crossed my mind on really bad calls, almost like a wave of nausea, when nothing I tried was working right, to throw up my hands and say "I can't do it." But I keep my head down, my face composed and I ruthlessly prioritize. Try this, keep trying that, try plan b, never give up, never stop thinking, slow down if you have to.

There's never been a perfect run. In hindsight there's always something I could have done faster, figured out sooner, something I left out, something I could have done a better way. It's upsetting for lay people to hear that everything does not go perfectly in emergencies, but that's what "emergency" means. Something fucked up. A motor vehicle collision is an accident.

You're better off not being in an ambulance. If you're going to have a motor vehicle accident, you shouldn't eat for 24 hours before. If you need to be intubated because your breathing is not supporting life, you're better off having it done by an anesthesiologist in a fully equipped surgical suite, rather than on your living room floor, on the grass by your backyard swing set, or on an asphalt road, by a 22 year old kid in muddy boots and a fireman's uniform, who might be doing it for the first time.

"Well, everyone has to have a first patient, so he can learn IVs," as the nurse told my first practice patient.

"Well, yeah, but I don't see why it has to be me."

My runs are good. I take pride in the outcomes and the process. I've saved a lot of lives and I haven't killed anyone yet. Someday I will. Everyone makes mistakes.

What I was going to talk about though was death. We see a lot of bodies. We get used to handling them. I've only had one person die under my hands, but I've found many dead people whom I could not resuscitate. Many of the patients I've brought to hospitals have died, some in short order, and some who were circling the drain in my box. Old people, people in the prime of life, kids, teenage suicides. The dismembered and the decomposed. In a later chapter, I'll talk about how the constant presence of death affects a person who, off shift, lives in the same safe, comfortable world as people with other jobs, but today I want to talk about two very beautiful deaths.

We responded, lights and sirens, code 3 as always, to a neat brick house in a rural community, carrying our bags across a well-manicured lawn and very conventional flower garden to a 50ish gentleman who answered the door. He led us to a sunny, immaculate little bedroom viewing the pecan trees through lace curtains.

"My mother lives here alone," he said. "She didn't answer her phone so I came by..." He stopped. He was calm though. "She's 98 years old."

A neatly made, single bed with a hand knit counterpane showed a few mounds and ridges arranged so an observant eye was persuaded to look further. I gently pulled back the cover, knowing what I would find.

She looked peaceful. Pale soft skin. Slender, composed. She had folded her arms over her breast, laid herself out. She had felt my Companion coming, my Enemy, my Boss, and, not wanting to give any trouble, got into her bed, barely ruffling the counterpane, pulled the covers over her head, crossed her arms and waited. There was no smell, no leaking bodily fluids.

I gently attached the leads of my cardiac monitor to her chest and belly, recorded asystole in two leads, lifted her shoulder and noted the dependent lividity, softly peeled back an eye and shined my penlight into her blown pupil. We all have our rituals.

Mine are the ones my society decrees are suited for death. Many are brought to a final resting place not in a chariot or hearse, but in my box to a gleaming hospital. In this case, I pronounced and called SO, a sheriff's officer, to vigil until the coroner arrived. He's in no hurry, nor need he be. I sat at a coffee table in the living room and wrote out my run form while I waited for SO. My most used medical instrument is a ballpoint pen.

That was the same week the Pope died. The newspapers went on and on about what a beautiful death he had achieved. The pomp and the circumstance.

He wasn't in the same class as this lady. Even by the standards of his own faith, hers had greater humility. And it wasn't her job to die well.

"She was a good Christian woman," her son said. It pissed me off. My stepfather is Jewish, my sister in law Hindu, and my mother an atheist. I didn't say anything.

We reported to SO, handed him a copy of the run form, cleared and took the next call. I'd like to be inspirational once in a while, make readers feel good if I can, but death is very rarely beautiful. One look tells us what the monitor confirms. The corpse stinks. Flesh is not flesh anymore but some alien putty rendered by a poor sculptor without respect for life. Death is a tragedy, whether some young person cut off before his life was run, a mourned and needed parent, or an old person whose body has gradually become more loathly and feebler and more decrepit until it stops working altogether. We meet Him all the time. He's part of our family. We don't respect him. His works don't freeze or awe us. We fight. We put our hands on his product, examine it without flinching, forget it without a second thought. But over time he wins. The average paramedic career is 5 to 8 years.

In the short term, though, we win. Even the most exquisite physicians eventually lose all their patients, but our patients die in hospitals, not in our box. Or they die at home, but death has fled the scene before we arrive to fight. Really, the full arrest is the only sport we usually lose. The other forms of combat we almost invariably win. We bring 'em in alive.

We took a call for respiratory distress. An ordinary suburban home. Inside too much furniture, a lifetime's, order and cleanliness admirably attempted but not entirely achieved by an elderly couple. The gentleman answered the door. He was slow, not only in gait. He told us his wife had been sick for a few days, and he had decided he ought to call us. He sounded apologetic, not quite sure of his ground.

In the bedroom on a double bed we found a thin, frail, elderly woman, probably less than a hundred pounds, "not even a dime," in EMT speech. People weighing more than 300 are called "lift assists" whether or not they're patients. Dusty but orderly bedroom. Her work, since her husband was not mentally up to living alone.

She was breathing rapidly. Moving air well, not really labored, but at 36 breaths a minute, where 12 to 20 is normal. She was extremely fragile and weak, and had been for a while, judging by her physique. Failure to thrive. Vital signs normal. No pain.

I asked her how she felt. Her voice was so soft I couldn't hear it, even in the quiet room. I bent my ear down to her mouth.

"I'm OK," she said.

She was not OK. Old people who breathe like someone still not fully recovered from a wind sprint are ominous. Especially if there's no apparent cause, no asthmatic wheezing, no burbling rhonchi from congestive heart failure, no cough or green sputum, no chest pain.

We couldn't get our stretcher into the bedroom, so I picked her up in my arms, under the knees and shoulders, and carried her out. We secured her to our stretcher. We ran lights and sirens to the nearest hospital while I started an IV and called it in to the emergency room. Starting lines in a moving ambulance, especially landing a difficult stick, is as much fun as it usually gets, up to darting people's chests or intubating. The country medics call them "rodeo sticks." I stuck in route on every call. The emergent ones required it—you don't delay transport for IVs except in cases where emergent IV meds are required even before transport. The non-emergent ones were for practice, I say. Actually for the same reason barflies enjoy landing darts in the center of the dartboard. Generally trauma requires ten minutes on scene—the "platinum ten minutes"—and no more than an hour—the "golden hour"-- between the trauma and definitive interventions in the hospital. Research and experience show people's systems can maintain for an hour or so even after very serious trauma. After that, they need repair. So for us, it's ABCD: Airway, Breathing , Circulation (including vitals), Diesel. Load and go. But in cervical collars and on backboards. There are exceptions.

Medical calls can be "stay and play." A full arrest takes at least half an hour on scene. You don't want to interrupt chest compressions for transport, and we carry everything the Emergency Department uses first line. Asthmatics and COPDers get nebulization. Lethal arrhythmias get IV drugs and shocks. CHFers get a whole cocktail. Chronic Obstructive Pulmonary Disease. Congestive Heart Failure. Supraventricular tachycardia.

No change in route.

"How are we doing? Does anything hurt?"

"I'm OK." Mouse voice.

The ED doc was even more pessimistic than I had been. He immediately began asking her husband about their wishes concerning Do Not Resuscitate. Did he want her to survive unconscious on a mechanical ventilator? Etc. Quite a shock to the poor old fellow.

She sat up in the bed, parchment skinned, breathing breathing breathing, a small crowd of staff around her in the trauma room.

"What's her mental status, anyway?" the doc asked me.

"She's fully alert and oriented, sir. GCS 15. She lives independently, fully ambulatory." 100 % on the Glasgow Coma Score. Just like you and me.

"Really," he said.

We rarely hear the end of the story. I prefer ambulance work to Air Life because at least we get the beginning and the context—people's lives and homes—plus we see a greater variety, a lot of medical, not just traumatic catastrophes. There are trauma junkies who relish every lascivious detail—all of us will recount luscious horrors you couldn't show on TV—but really trauma is all the same. Stop the bleeding, collar and board, lights and sirens, IV en route. Medical calls are more interesting. Is your patient unresponsive because of his low sugar, his cardiac rhythm, breathing problems, an MI, choking, seizure, stroke? All requiring different interventions, some multiple. But we still rarely hear the outcome. You used to be able to call an ER nurse you knew, but now it's a HIPPA violation for her to tell you anything once you've transferred care. You could keep the patient's phone number, I guess. I never have. Seems intrusive. And by then new cases have come and gone.

Having grown up on modernist and post-modernist fiction, Heisenberg uncertainty principles, Rashomon, relativity, modern skepticism about the accuracy of individual or even collective perception, I've been almost pleased with this state of affairs. I regard it as pure realism when compared to stories, "arced" or not. "What is truth?" said Nietzsche's favorite New Testament character. Besides, I lose interest after 15 minutes.

In this case, however, I happened to bring another patient into the same emergency room a few hours later. After I handed in my paperwork, I peeked behind the curtains into the bay where I'd left my elderly lady. She was sitting up, looking about the same as when I'd left her, and as when I'd found her. But she wasn't breathing anymore.

Husband not in evidence.

I stopped the ER doc to ask him what she had died of. Normally I won't address one unless spoken to first or giving report, unlike RNs. You chat and joke with them.

"Respiratory failure."

Well, duh.

"Do you know what caused it?" Persistent, because I was interested in this one.

"Her blood gases were way off." He didn't feel like talking about it. Why, I don't know. All this added was that, while she was ventilating adequately, cellular respiration was not adequate. Air was going in and out but it wasn't being used. What I had surmised 40 seconds into my exam.

She had struck a chord, skinny little thing with her whispery alert voice. A home maker. I had been the last person to put my arms around her. Carried her to her final rest. Her last intimacy. Angel of death.

It wears on you.

FYI

Perhaps you would like to know in more detail how we work the assessment on scene of a patient like this lady. If not, skip on to the next chapter.

After we get the call, as described in the first chapter, we have 2 minutes to get rolling, and we proceed to the address, lights and sirens no matter what the call. In this case we were toned out for a "sick person." That doesn't tell us much, but we never know what we are going to find anyway. If it's a gunshot wound, stabbing, assault, suicide or other psych call, we stage near the address but out of sight until a sheriff's officer has cleared the scene.

For this call we rolled up to an older brick house in a decent, inexpensive older neighborhood. All this is not scene setting. It begins to tell us what we can expect and what to watch out for. The lawn and garden were nice, respectable, but not kept up really well. The old gentleman I described met us at the door. Old, worn but clean clothes. His house had too much furniture, was dusty, but orderly and picked up. Again, gives us an idea of what kind of people live here, their competence, energy level, likely compliance with drug regimens, scrupulosity about health care, their smoking, alcoholism or drug abuse.

He didn't seem panicky or in a hurry. We followed him to the bedroom. The lady described above was on the bed. She was frail, elderly, breathing as described. She was looking at me alertly and her face seemed controlled and alert, no Alzheimer type rigidity or slackness.

My partner took vitals, which were all normal except the rate of breathing, and interviewed the husband further, gathering her meds and insurance and demographic data along the way. I interviewed and examined the patient, as described, and noted that she had clear lungs, good oxygen saturation, was alert and oriented, had good skin color and tone, did not appear grievously sick, though obviously quite ill. By that I mean that she was not gasping or covered with sweat or in obvious pain. It's hard to describe. You look at someone and form an idea of how sick they are, subject to revision.

What I gathered was that this did not seem like an MI. No fainting spells, no chest pain, back pain or radiating pain. No nausea, no diaphoresis, normal EKG. She was having breathing problems obviously but albuterol didn't seem like a good idea. Respiratory therapists seem to think albuterol inhalers are good for everyone but albuterol does strain your heart a little by raising your heart rate and it's mostly for opening up airways and alveoli, which did not sound like this lady's problem. I did not hear burbly rhonchi, indicating water in her lungs, she had no edema, no history that I could ascertain of heart disease, so congestive heart failure was also unlikely, and that meant that giving her a diuretic like Lasix, or giving her nitroglycerine to open up some vascular space for the excess water, was not indicated. There was no congestion. You can't hear pneumonia much of the time but I did not hear crackles anywhere and she had no fever, and did not appear sick in that way, so pneumonia was possible but not likely. Anyway we don't do anything for that except transport more rapidly. Pulmonary embolism was another possibility, but she was not laboring to breathe, and she had few risk factors, as she had not been injured or had recent surgery or been bedbound. Nor was she obese, and the low oxygen sats or low blood pressure which sometimes come with a PE were also absent. So my conclusion was that there was something seriously metabolically wrong, organ failure, failure to thrive. It could easily involve her heart, but did not seem to be an arrhythmia or MI, based on our 12 lead EKG.

I'm trying to show you what our decision making process is like. Perhaps in too much detail. We can't make a diagnosis, except a provisional, rule out X one, and for many of the conditions we find, we can't do anything except transport. But often there is an appropriate, useful intervention we can perform, and even if not, I like to know what's going on as best I can, just out of curiously, but also because it helps me answer questions in the ER, and gives me a leg up if something else happens en route. I know where I am.

4 NASTY CALLS

The question I hear most is "what's the worst thing you've ever seen?" or "what's the worst call you ever had?" People don't mean the one which caused me the most stress or was hardest to run or had the worst outcome or got me into the most trouble. My service employed 3 people whose job it was to hunt and fire medics. They were good at their job in the sense they caused a lot of turnover, but poor at weeding out bad medics. Their hits were more random than lightening. Bad medics, mediocre medics, and also 5 of the 6 best medics I ever met. And the turnover in their own ranks was so great that 3 or 4 people served in each position during the five years I worked there, guaranteeing that they had no way of knowing, really, who the good people were, who had made a mistake versus who habitually made mistakes. They just picked out run forms with unfashionable errors, or perceived errors, the flavor of the week, and did their best to entrap and prosecute, rather than educate or evaluate, which is what Control of Quality Investigations are supposed to do. One month it would be signed refusals, another month nonprotocoled medics starting IVs. The one thing they did guarantee was that training and reeducation expenses remained exorbitant, and that a majority of the field medics were inexperienced. At five years "in the county" I was the second longest serving medic on a 911 post.

I went on trial probably yearly. When their doc was involved I'd walk. He was cold as ice, at best referred to me as "a valuable resource," somewhere between a pulse oximeter and a cardiac monitor, but he had a lot of common sense, and knew a lot of emergency medicine. Though you'd always take a hit, like the IRS. It was usually retraining, which for me was kind of like throwing Brer Rabbit into the briar patch. "I was born and bred in the briar patch." I love training.

What people mean is what was the nastiest and ugliest call, the most disgusting gore, I ever saw. Stuff most medics actually love to talk about, at least among themselves.

So if you'll join me for a moment in my prurient interests I'll tell you a couple. This is the chapter you might want to skip if you have weak stomach or a sense of personal dignity. But I will leave out the really wrenching stories, the true worst calls, for the burn out chapter. They're beyond prurient interest. They're the ones that come back to you at night on your days off, though I won't say anything ever interrupted me getting as much sleep as I could. I can and have slept bolt upright in an ambulance running hot to a distant call, 90 miles away, to take a kid from a local ER to a Pediatric hospital on a day nothing could fly.

We took a call for a train v ped one evening. That is, train vs pedestrian. You never know. It could be a false alarm, or someone bumping his head on an exit stair, but pedestrians don't usually do well against trains. MV ped is bad enough. In fact much of our practice and protocols comes from the epidemic of trauma in the 50s and 60s which led to the invention of EMS. The first crews used hearses, by legend dumping the corpse in a convenient hidden spot to be picked up later, after they dealt with the emergency. An old medic told me they used to chuck the victim in the back, speed to the hospital and then, after checking the contents, either turn left to the morgue or right to the emergency room.

Then crews learned to backboard against spinal cord injuries, extricate, bandage, splint, tourniquet. It got so they were delivering exquisitely wrapped corpses to the ER, since the statistics hadn't improved since the hearse days. In fact got worse.

Then they invented the "golden hour" between trauma and definitive care, the "platinum ten minutes" you were supposed to be on scene, the triage protocol ABCD. Airway Breathing Circulation Diesel. About the platinum ten minutes, the most experienced medic in our class told us, "The main thing, it ain't gonna happen." You're lucky to roll in 20.

Still between that and the airbags, seat belts, crumple zones, improved highways, sandbagged pillars, side impact beams, it got so you arrived at horrendous wrecks to find everyone walking around. Unless it was semi vs car, or a motorcycle, or someone had forgotten his seatbelt. But we still kept the old protocols. Deformed steering wheels had to be reported. They used to mean someone had taken a battering ram in the chest. Now the little Toyota wheel will be found dangling, without having hit anything except the airbag.

Train v ped though. Still bad. We had trouble accessing the scene. Railroad tracks are not fully accessible by ambulance. We found the right service road, pushing pushing pushing to get there. Always pushing pushing pushing to get the medic (me) in the back of a rolling ambulance with the patient. Turned out we were tromping through the ragweed on the wrong side of the track, with the train between us and the patient. We crawled over a coupling. Now we could get to the patient, but how would we get the patient to the ambulance? Train crew showed up and said they would uncouple and pull the train up a few yards.

The body was between the tracks, initially under the train. The head though was five or six feet away, lying on the cinder like a bowling ball. It was looking at us. No particular expression.

My partner said, "I really don't need to see a lot more stuff like this in my life."

Not much blood. It really didn't bother me much at the time. Even later, except cumulatively, it didn't have much impact. I was relieved. Injured people I must save, quickly and adeptly, pushing pushing pushing. Dead people aren't my job. This one didn't even need to have a cardiac monitor on him. Didn't have to check for dependent lividity or pupillary reflexes. A true decapitation is pronounceable per se. San Antonio Fire once left a motor vehicle accident victim on scene with the requisite yellow blanket over her when she was still alive. Even though a cop said she was still breathing. And that's how the coroner found her two hours later. We joked that SAFD's new motto was "we got you covered." They had found brain matter on the dashboard. So I put a monitor on everyone, except the two cases in this chapter.

We were more worried about the train engineer. In a previous case the engineer had to be transported with instant PTSD.

This one was taking it in stride. Hyper of course. It was his second. The victim had never moved from his position on the track, even with the horn blaring and brakes screaming.

We considered and dismissed suicide. Even a determined suicide would have at least flinched. The lack of blood also indicated he was probably dead already.

The engineer said he'd seen a car's headlights waiting by the tracks. A deserted location, he'd assumed one of the managers was checking his speed, until he saw the body.

A gang hit, we decided. Mexican mafia. South San Antonio. They had killed him already and were making some kind of statement.

We cleared and took our next call. No matter what they are, you just go on, take the next call. I had a bizarre impulse to pick up the head by the hair and bring it along, like Evelyn Waugh's "coconut." As a souvenir, as in his war novel? To a hospital? Just one of these nightmarish flashes passing through the brain like heat lightning.

We took a 3 AM call for a hang-up in the old German farm country even farther southwest, a deserted rural road with a few decrepit houses widely spread. Fields, brush, weeds. The caller had dialed 911 and hung up. When dispatch called the number back, the phone was picked up and hung up again, several times. In the old days, before caller ID, panicky callers would reply to queries about their address with "never mind that. Just hurry over here." "Hurry over WHERE?" the dispatcher would persist, patiently. The protocol for hang ups is SO—sheriff's officer—checks it out first. We stage nearby, waiting for his instructions. The cops walk into these things alone, with just their equipment and radio. Scenes considered too dangerous for a crew of brave fireman or pairs of heroic medics or all of the above.

Cliff parked the ambulance about a half mile east of the address. He was talking on the county radio to the firemen first responders. They were staged a half mile west of the address. No way of knowing how long before SO showed up.

Cliff, incurably gregarious, decided it would be much nicer to stage with the fireman and catch up on things with them while we waited. One of our few disagreements was over his propensity to hang out at bullshit calls or nonemergent transports to chat, when I wanted to get the patient going. Never know when one will crash. It's never any fun trying to explain why you were on scene so long. He also liked to schmooze at the hospital afterward instead of going back to the station to nap.

"OK," I said sleepily, my mind on other things. "Hey, wait a minute. If we're east of the address and Fire is west of it, won't we be going right by the house if we…." Too late. We peered at it on the way by. Dark. Old. Built by ranchers who could build anything. Though maybe not as well as professionals.

Cliff was visiting happily with the fireman and I was napping when SO sped by, lights flashing blue and red in the humid dark. No city light, no moon. Hackberry trees dusty in our running lights. Better than a movie. All we needed was Ry Cooder. The officer pulled up to the house, knocked on the door. Someone admitted him. Cliff had thus, you can gather, crept the ambulance closer to the scene again. Curiosity killed the medic. Cliff was fucking fearless. The best partner I ever head, a true gentleman in tact and sensitivity, vastly experienced and carrying me through my newbie year, a great single father, funny as hell, but also a menace to life and limb, and as conservative in mores as they come. The N word signified another race of people to him, in all sincerity. And yet the kindest, most considerate person you could meet. Particularly fullspeed when it came to helping children. When we did a birth, I let him do the delivery on the trailer floor while I only supervised and made suggestions. He loved it. Taking Mom and baby to the hospital afterwards too. Childbirth is a Basic skill, believe it or not. Until Mom or baby crash.

"Yes, ma'am. If you were in the hospital, an obstetrician with ten years' experience of hundreds of deliveries, 4 years of medical school, 6 years of residency and a staff of pros would be helping you. But don't worry. I read that chapter very carefully. And I did pass my GED, no matter what they say."

Cliff was a peerless mimic too. We had one ODS (On Duty Supervisor) who was gay and had an odd voice. His nickname was Skeeter, if that gives you an idea. Mosquito. Cliff could do him perfectly. Cliff called up Skeeter's following shift ODS once.

"Jack," he said, "how you doing?"

"Ah, okay. What's up, Skeeter?"

"Did I leave a black notebook there? It would be on the file cabinet."

"No, I don't see anything. Could it be somewhere else?"

"Na, don't worry about it. Maybe I left it at my mom's house."

"Well OK then. Hope you find it."

"Uh, Jack?"

"Yeah?"

"Jack, what are you wearing?"

There was a momentary stunned and appalled silence, then

"Cliff, is that you?" Jack sounded mad as hell, and he was Cliff's boss. Cliff hung up.

The cop wasn't in the house more than a minute before we heard a gunshot. Oh Jesus, we thought, what do we do about this? We figured the cop had been hit. Call more cops? We're unarmed and not trained or permitted to act as police officers, but our trained instinct is to help a brother officer any way we can. At a mass casualty incident we take care of our own first. By protocol. A lightly injured cop gets our attention before a seriously wounded citizen, in reverse of standard triage. Because it inhibits and demoralizes responders to feel no one has their back.

Cliff headed for the house with the handheld radio. I pulled the ambulance up. The firemen eventually followed Cliff. I was now honorbound to rescue Cliff if need be, but I wasn't looking forward to it.

Second gunshot. But I also hear people trooping out the back of the house, making the inimitable racket of firemen. I sit in the ambulance. I cruise it slowly toward where I imagine the back can be reached. Dead end. I don't really know what to do.

I key up the radio and say "203 203 direct." When you call another truck directly, letting them know where to find an address, or something they need to know about a patient, you say "203 207 direct," i.e. not via dispatch. This is done sparingly, and you keep it short. With one radio band, you don't want a lot of trucks clogging up the line chatting with each other. In fact everything is kept short. If you have more to say or something you don't want everyone in the county to know, you say "standby for public service," which means you're going to call your interlocutor on the telephone. A language and customs all their own.

Cliff had the handheld and I had the truck radio so I didn't know any other way to find out where he was. This was before cell phones.

"203 203 direct."

Everyone listens to what everyone else is doing, follows all the other trucks around via radio traffic, so by now the entire county was rapt. "What the hell were you guys up to?" they all asked later.

"203," said Cliff.

"Where are you and how do I get there?"

"Come down the little dirt road just west of the house."

There didn't seem to be any dirt road west of the house, little or big, but I wasn't going to make any more of a fool of myself on the radio, calling my own unit number. I drove across some firm looking grass and along a kind of caliche driveway cum wash. Pretty soon I saw flashlights.

I stopped the ambulance, left it running, got out and locked it. Hiked up the creek bed or whatever it was. 4 wheel drive trail. Cliff and the firemen came over to lead me to the right spot. They all tended to be solicitous of me due to my advanced age and small experience and due to the fact that fire, police and EMS bond. It's a fraternity. On the job, people really do watch your back. Except the backstabbers.

We all trooped over to a stony ditch lit by numerous powerful flashlights, full of tall weeds and a body. He was crashed into the side of the ditch. Obese, ugly, fair skinned, out of shape. He may have died young but he did not leave a beautiful corpse. The high powered hunting rifle he had used was already gathered up by the cop for evidence. I contemplated putting a monitor on him, but once again this was one of the few times when it was unnecessary. He had blown off the entire top of his head from the cheekbones up. You could look into his skull pan and see what was left of his pink brains. The rest were scattered around the ditch.

The story was he had been feeling depressed for a long time. Living at home, unemployed, with his parents. They had heard him leave the house earlier. Upon investigation they had found the rifle missing. Soon after that they saw an ambulance cruise by. A while later the sheriff's officer showed up and the rest is as above.

We heard later that the first shot had gone into his chest. Still alive, he had finished the job with the head shot. Kind of an honorable death in a way. He hadn't left a mess in his house, hadn't left the body for his parents to find, and had shown tremendous determination and grit finishing the job. Git er done. This was no gesture, no botched attempt.

Though the corpse was still hideous. An appalling thing to see at 4 AM in dark hardscrabble country. 300 lbs. of dismembered human pig. No helping that though, really. Corpses. The final hurdle that would keep me from ever committing suicide, even after imagining my children's feelings, is my commitment to saving life, not rendering it into meat, but pulling it back into life. It's a matter of respect, an oath. Though that's easy for me to say. Unless you've actually done it, you can't really put yourself in his mind to judge.

Still, a course of antidepressants and some counseling would have been my recommendation, and who's to say that wouldn't have worked?

We took an MV ped at the S bend on I35 we called dead man's curve because at least once a year, before TXDOT finally put in barriers, a semi would miss the turn and pile into whatever was handy. We'd arrive to find the semi on its side, big as a house, and the driver walking around unhurt, talking on the phone to his boss. Anything he had hit was demolished, houses, cars, trees, railings, human beings.

But this time it was an SUV with a dented bumper and a shattered windshield pulled over near a 30ish, dirty, poorly dressed man whose upper body was supine and lower body prone. Where the twist was, a heap of bowels spilled out onto the interstate. Had this been a suicide? A mishap while crossing? Someone under the influence? We pronounced, called it in and cleared. It took me a while to explain it to the doc. He wasn't really following my description.

I did put the monitor on this one. No heart rhythm, not surprisingly. I considered later whether it would have been possible to cover the bowels in wet dressings, twist the body onto a backboard somehow and transport, had his heart still been going. It was hard to imagine. Delivering this reeking twisted corpse to an emergency room. I would have had to travel with it, try to start an IV and the like, but at least cleaning up the ambulance would have been Cliff's chore.

5 STUPIC PET TRICKS

One of the hitches with universal health care is that a majority of the people who have serious health problems either brought them on themselves or exacerbated their conditions by their own actions or inactions, and the same is true for trauma. There's a psychological component to their management of most of their conditions even when the condition is not purely psychological to start with. Eugenics has gotten a bad name, and rightly so, since it would be so difficult to apply, Bach being the 14th son of a syphilitic and all that (OK, maybe the facts are wrong, but the point is valid). Still you have to wonder whether we are managing our gene pool, not by encouraging the most capable to breed, but the exact opposite. We are saving the lives of people who, evolutionarily considered, maybe shouldn't multiply.

It sometimes seems to me that in the future every third vehicle will be an ambulance, transporting every fifth person.

I wonder how many percent of the population could pass my 24 hour test. Set them gently under a shade tree on a clement day, return the next day to see if they survived, without ventilators, insulin, oxygen, air conditioning, wheel chairs, dialysis, medications.

I've walked into hospital rooms to find an entire clan camped around gramaw's bed. She's comatose on a ventilator, fed via peg tube, blood pressure maintained by dopamine drip. The family, medically ignorant, is sure gramaw is still in there. She used to cook and keep house for them; in this particular stage of life she lies in a hospital bed with no pupillary reflexes, at a cost of hundreds of thousands a year. Meanwhile my partner can't get insurance for his mildly asthmatic 2 year old son, otherwise perfectly normal, who may even outgrow his condition. This is not triage as we are taught it in EMT Basic. Which I think everyone should take in high school. Leave out the equipment training, and just teach some basic anatomy and physiology, what to do in common emergencies, and how to take care of yourself.

We wouldn't go on scene to find a 50 year. old woman, visiting relatives for Thanksgiving, with a blood pressure of 80/40, semi-conscious. She had been told to take her new BP med before bedtime, so, staying up late for Thanksgiving, figured 10 pm was about right. The med knocked her flat, more or less as it's supposed to, and we find her seated, with her relatives holding her head up, trying to drain all the blood out, as they follow the correct procedure for a neck injury. We lay her down, put her feet up. Fixed. Still, she gets fluid and goes to the ER just in case. Not going to leave a patient presenting with an 80 systolic on scene.

Or consider the household flooded in the 9th ward by Katrina. Only one inhabitant was employed, and him only part time, as a roofer. When the first floor flooded they moved to the second, then the third and finally the attic. Fortunately this was where he stored his tools. He broke through to the roof, pulled mama up out of her wheelchair, levered 400 lb. uncle up somehow, his diabetic one legged wife, and a couple toddlers, and there they all sat, awaiting rescuers. Not enough rescuers.

400 pounders, 500, 600. We took an 840 lb. guy to the hospital once. Took three crews. He lived in his converted garage, as access through doors no longer possible. On a bed with casters. We unscrewed the antlers from the ambulance

floor, and left them behind, with the stretcher they normally secured. We pulled his bed down the driveway. Caster wheel tore right off. We rolled and levered him onto a specially made vinyl pull sheet. Three medics on one side, three on the other. One of the handles tore right off. We pulled him into the ambulance onto the floor. Propped his head and back up on pillows because the morbidly obese can't breathe lying flat. They move around on scooters because they're too fat to walk; are on ventilators because they're too fat to breathe.

Once they're bedbound or even housebound, you figure if someone stops feeding them, they must lose weight. Enablers sometimes, but we had a 400 lber who kept asking for food the entire ambulance ride. True, her short term memory wasn't working, but, "Would you have a little piece of cheese?"

"No ma'am we don't carry food in the ambulance. It's not permitted by the department of health."

"OK." Two minutes.

"Would you perhaps have a soft drink? I'm thirsty."

"No ma'am, we don't carry....'

"OK." Two minutes.

"Could I maybe get a cracker?"

"No ma'am, we don't carry...."

"Sir, could I...." After 35 minutes of this my partner was ready to put anything into her mouth just to shut her up. My new partner, a 240 lb. body builder with anger management problems. Big old scars on his knuckles. Leonine Egyptian head. Nurses walked into doors looking at him. Sudden deep sighs. Generally I handled him very carefully. He was a huge amount of help on scene. The 260 lb. patient who faked seizures he carried easily down her trailer's rickety homemade steps ("I don't think you can fix that with duct tape"), which usually took 8 firemen and substantial negotiation, physical and moral. Still, on slow shifts, being as I'm a hero who likes to live dangerously, and, by the evidence, not a guy who always acts in his own best interest, I'd hand him a pair of small gloves when he was distracted by his patient. Watched him struggle to pull them on, until he realized what was wrong. He elected to find that funny, but it was a near thing.

One morning at 6:45, just ten minutes before my relief usually shows up, I got toned out for a full arrest. We arrived, walked in a door opened by a remarkably calm, 40ish, well dressed Hispanic woman. She indicated her mother, who was sitting up in a bed in the living room. People who are "not breathing" often turn out to be not only alive but even in glowing health, perhaps merely asleep, or post ictal after a seizure, but this lady was stone cold dead, blue. She was sitting up because, at 650 lbs., the human inner tube around her propped her up like a kid's punching doll.

Jesus, I thought. How am I going to get her off the bed? How am I going to intubate her? Find a vein for IV access? Do chest compressions? Ventilate her supine, when she can't breathe in that position even normally? And I was going to do my very utmost to do all of these, if necessary. NOT TRY, DO. Failure is not acceptable, even when it's inevitable.

I crawled onto her extra wide bed, not considering until later that I was wading in urine. Much more important considerations at hand. You screen out or remove the inessential. I lift the cover to find a billow of flesh. I'm not sure what part of her body this is, but I raise the edge of it to find a magenta stain of dependent lividity. Once the blood has pooled it can no longer be circulated. If it could, it would be so toxic it would kill the patient all over again. Dependent lividity. I can pronounce. Thank you, God. Thank you.

The morbidly obese realize fat is not good for their health, though perhaps they don't realize they WILL have serious health problems starting no later than 40, perhaps including death. But they don't realize their medical care will be compromised too. You can't find veins, you can't move them to the hospital quickly, you can't hear their lungs, you can't get to their organs with a scalpel, you can't intubate, you can't palpate. The body has great redundancies, like aircraft. The heart can support more than one person. Until it starts to age. Then enough insulin production for one person is not enough for two or three, by weight. But clearly the obese can't help it, since no one really wants to be fat. Meanwhile the mythology grows. We're genetically programmed to love MacDonald's. (Soggy white bread with poor quality meat?) Healthy food is expensive. (Rice and beans? Then why are sub-Saharan Africans and Pakistanis skinny?) It's a strange mystery. But it does leave a poor impression of human beings' rationality.

We respond to a guy who has unscrewed his radiator cap while his engine is still hot. I was taught not to do this even before I really knew what a radiator was, and a good decade before I even drove. I think people are genetically programmed not to do this. They remember it even if they have Alzheimer's and can't remember their names.

But the guy only has some 1st degree burns on his torso—no more than a bad sunburn--because he put on his safety glasses and bent out of the way best he could. He saved his eyesight and face. We rinsed him off. Rinse burns with cool running water for ten minutes. And then we took a signed refusal. Even I wasn't going to transport someone for sunburn.

But think about this for a minute. Why did he put on the safety glasses and bend out of the way? Because he knew unscrewing the cap might vent live steam? Then why did he unscrew the cap? Because he figured it was OK to fry his torso, so long as his head was safe?

We answer a call for a 30 year old male who has had a seizure while tiling a roof. The reason the roof was being tiled was because a month before a car had missed the curve the house was on, slammed into it, and exploded, burning it to the ground. The residents of the house got out, but nobody could extricate the occupants of the car. Bystanders and an EMT crew listened to them scream as they burned to death. Fire didn't make it in time.

I climbed up the ladder, still in place. It's a shallow roof, but Cliff is worried about me. I'm spryer than I look though. The roofer is lying up there on his back. Fortunately it's not summer, so it's not unbearably hot on the tile.

"Hey, buddy, how you doing?

"Head hurts." He still looks kind of dopey but I gather, ABC, that his airway is patent, since he can talk. ("I can't breathe I can't breathe" can mean many dire things, but not that the patient isn't breathing. Screaming babies are healthy babies.) The roofer's muscle tone is good, he's holding up his head to look at me, he's answering sensibly, his color is OK, and, given he's focusing his eyes on me, I don't need to check his pupils yet, if at all. No visible injuries, no blood, no mechanism of injury. He's still ON the roof.

"You had a seizure, huh?"

"I guess so."

He can't really know for sure of course: you don't know you're unconscious. That's what unconscious means. So asking someone if they lost consciousness is pointless. Let them describe the accident, see if they have antero or retrograde amnesia. So his answer means, instead, that he's had one before. It's not a new thing. He's still post ictal—the dopey or semi-conscious period after a seizure--but he's recovering. Most seizure calls, the seizure is over by the time you get there. Most people who seize while you're there are faking. If they don't piss themselves, aren't good actors, or are able to respond during or after in any purposive way, those are more clues it's a pseudoseizure. Not definitive though. People have partial seizures and fake major ones. Piss themselves on purpose. They get valium just the same. I won't say they earned it, but anyone going to these lengths to get a dose of benzo, gets one. Because you can't tell for sure.

And there is status epilepticus, where a person either seizes again without recovering, or keeps seizing. Since you don't usually breathe when you're seizing, this is life threatening. You gain venous access, by force majeure if necessary, and shoot valium into them. Even for absence seizures, where they're suddenly not home.

I've had those, and had a frequent flyer, an FLK as pediatricians call it--funny looking kid with a genetic abnormality—who was still seizing despite his parents' rectal valium. He was about 6 or 8 but looked 2, kind of toddler pudgy. An impossible stick, until I noticed some weird veins wandering across his chest. Managed to get a small needle in one while we were flying to the hospital, and damn if the little devil doesn't reach down a chubby hand and yank it out. Still seizing.

Normally they're tachycardic too. You might expect a slow heart rate, given how dopey they still are, but their body is making up for the huge effort, akin to all in wrestling.

I'm taking pulse and blood pressure, pulse oximetry, while I'm talking to the roofer. Cliff is looking up the ladder, following the action. By now I'm sitting, feet tripoded downhill.

"So you have a seizure disorder? Do you take medicine for it?"

"Naw, it's too expensive."

"Probably cheaper than falling off a roof though."

"Well, I only have about one a year."

"Hmm. Try not to have one while you're swimming, or in the bath tub, or crossing the street, or driving, or on a roof pitched steeper than this one. Plus they can damage your brain further, and they get worse."

He got the point. He knows he can't choose when he's going to have one. And while I spend little time on roofs, he's a roofer. So he's my poster boy for this chapter. I considered calling it "The Epileptic Roofer." But insight never cured anything but ignorance. Sometimes that's enough, but being smart doesn't make you rich or famous. Not even rich enough to afford Dilantin, the old tried and true seizure med. My advice and three bucks would buy him a day's supply. He gets a free ride to the emergency room if he wants one, and he doesn't have to pay his emergency room bill if his credit rating isn't a concern, but no one will give him Dilantin.

Pharmacies don't deliver in the US either. You can get a pizza or a motor vehicle delivered to your door, but not a 2 ounce bottle of pills. So if you're sick or handicapped or elderly or underage or have no car, you have to hope someone will drive to a pharmacy to fill your prescription for you. Otherwise, dial 911.

So who's not behaving intelligently here, the patients, or us?

6 BIG ANNIE

We had a frequent flyer who lived with her doting husband in a nearby trailer camp. I'll call her Big Annie. We got calls because her ankle hurt, possibly she broke it, because she didn't feel well, or because she was blue and barely breathing. She weighed a good 300 lbs. and was bedbound, paralyzed on one side by a stroke. I was young and earnest in the profession then, so I spent some time with her and her husband, explaining to them that if she didn't lose weight she was at increased risk for another stroke. Most medics and docs probably would've figured this was a waste of time. At a later stage in my career I might have figured they had given up, knowing one stroke follows another even in people of normal weight. Especially in diabetics and people with comorbid conditions, like her. The statistics even for a TIA, a transient ischemic incident (a stroke or cerebral artery block which clears up fully, usually rapidly) is that a full blown stroke usually follows within five years.

But they had not given up. At least in their own fashion. The husband walked up to me in the supermarket later, thanking me for all my help and good care. It took a while before I figured out who he was. I was touched. I felt I'd been kind of impatient, but apparently I'd only felt that way. I'd acted patient. I control my expressions pretty carefully on scene. Often only my partner knew. It would be a glance and a suppressed smile rather than rolling in the aisles holding our sides. You may be having a ball running a full arrest, but it's not going to be any fun for the relatives. You can't expect them to realize that you wouldn't be there doing a good job in those kind of conditions if you didn't enjoy your work. He said I'd explained everything no one had bothered to explain to them, like stroke risk factors. He said she was on a diet and had lost weight. By the time we saw her again, it wasn't apparent.

I'm sure they were trying, but there was a lot didn't meet the eye, for example the bushel basket of potatoes in the kitchen by the sink, and the way she pronounced the word gravy with trailer camp relish. Also, if she couldn't walk, what was the step stool by the sink for? How do you sprain your ankle in bed?

On scene you're focused on essentials, stripped down to move, so you don't contemplate all this stuff, unless you happen to be discussing it with another medic later.

It was always a huge hassle getting her out. Firemen don't really like touching patients. They're helpful, they're strong, they'll lift anything for you, but what they really like is structure fires. Even though 80% of their calls are "assist EMS." They block off motor vehicle wrecks, carry stretchers, "lift assist" 400 pounders who fell off their scooters while transferring to their beds, take vitals while waiting for us, whatever. This has come about historically because their equipment keeps getting more expensive, their manpower boosted, but the fires fewer, as people smoke less, heaters get safer and everything gets more fireproof. So rather than let them play basketball or polish their truck a third time, counties had the bright idea of training them to help us. Our calls do not get fewer.

They're really a joy to work with. Funny, goodnatured, gung ho. Unthinkingly brave. One of the NW guys used to park his red truck in our lot when he got behind in his payments, so repo couldn't find it. Moose at Northwest Fire claimed to be a graduate of the Culinary Institute. He prepared elaborate Thanksgiving and Christmas dinners for the crews who were on duty on those days. Holidays are busy. People get drunk and have lots of extra time to get in trouble. Very good food. Very much appreciated.

My favorite Moose story though is the day he came out to assist San Antonio EMS with a motor vehicle. They were in our territory because we had more victims than crew, what's called a mass casualty incident. An SAEMS medic was standing next to a wrecked sedan when Moose came over to help.

The medic said, "We need the jaws of life."

Moose said, "You mean you want the door open?"

"Yeah," the medic said impatiently. "Don't you carry it in your truck?"

"You mean you want the door open."

"Yeah, get the jaws." Moose does not look as bright as he is. The medic was glaring at him by now.

Moose grabbed the door handle, braced his feet, yanked it off its hinges and threw it in the gutter.

"What else?" he said.

Firemen were never in the least shy about using their strength. They'd pretty much demolish and drown houses with the axes and hoses. Big mirrors were a favorite. One was following a colleague of mine onto a chest pain scene with his axe once. She said, "What are you planning to do with that?" He looked sheepish and brought it back to his truck.

But they did not like touching patients. It's funny, I put my hands all over patients immediately, but I hate to touch them without gloves on. Feels creepy. When I notice reluctance in myself, even with gloves, it means I don't intuit them as sick or injured. The usual contact rules re-apply. I stab injured or sick kids with IVs without mercy, but if I think they're OK, I can't do it.

So it would be up to me to make the major effort of getting Big Annie from her corner bed in her narrow trailer, 300 lbs. of dead weight, onto the stretcher. "That's why you make the big bucks," the firemen would say if I bitched. It's a standard joke, made as often as appropriate, like "another life saved" for really trivial calls.

Annie had a habit of getting away from us. She usually wore only a thin nylon nighty which rode up to her shoulders the minute you made contact and, though her husband was very attached to her, bathing her was not among his best nursing skills. So I'd be on my knees on the floor pushing and lifting with all my might on the nether parts, the nighty around her neck, while a squeamish fireman or two gingerly pulled on her arms. My nose and face were inches, well, you get the picture. The firemen were vastly entertained, though they were professional enough not to stagger with laughter at my expense until later.

I had to put an oral airway into her gullet right on her scooter once. She presented blue and unconscious. The firemen helped me get her onto the stretcher efficiently that time. Wading in bodily fluids was always my job, lifting usually theirs. I bagged her with the bag valve mask and pure oxygen and gave her some atropine for her slow heart rate. By the time we got to Wilford Hall Medical Center she was alert and oriented, warm pink and dry. She was answering the doc's questions with the J tube still stuck down her throat. Military docs have this ability to male bond instantly with crew. It always felt warm in WHMC, not only physically in the trauma room.

"I've never seen anybody who could talk with one of those things in her throat," he said. She was still hard to understand, though, so he pulled it out. She didn't seem to have much of a gag reflex, if any. One of the firemen said he finally understood why her husband was so fond of her. They were routinely and unthinkingly obscene.

We were assigned to take her home once too. We had brought a patient to St Luke's, so Dispatch assigned us to bring her back from there to our neighborhood, on the way to our station, since our service was shorthanded that day. We didn't normally do non-emergent transports, so Cliff was already displeased. We took a substantial cut on hourly rate so we could dedicate ourselves to 911, and rest on standby when there were no calls. A necessity when you're on a 24 hour shift. You have to get sleep when you can.

So Cliff objected. He was lying in the back of the ambulance sulking. "I'm sorry I'm being such an asshole," he said after a while. It was really unlike him. "But we at least have to get lift assist." Besides being over 300 lbs., Annie had the unique ability I've described to slide and flop. She'd managed to sag to the floor in the middle of the Methodist ER once when Cliff and I and a nurse were attempting to move her from the stretcher to a wheelchair. She was offended they didn't offer her a bed.

I eventually came to the conclusion that she enjoyed sliding away from us. Some kind of substitute for hugs, perhaps. The reason I know is that Mack Cutter, playing On Duty Supervisor that day, finally had to come down to St Luke's to be lift assist. He was mad to start with, because they were shorthanded and overwhelmed with calls that day, which was why we were being asked to transport Annie home. He'd suggested we get someone at the hospital to lift assist, and get firemen at the other end. This might have worked and might not. Easy to say, hard to arrange. I'm sympathetic to management's problems when they're explained to me, and if I'm asked nicely, but it's not ingrained in my blue collar pay structure or working conditions to empathize spontaneously. It's not like they waste any sympathy on us. We are entitled to lift assist with patients over 300 lbs., even ones less slippery than Big Annie. And most of us eventually damage our backs anyway. And aren't upwardly mobile.

So Cutter shows up. "This is bullshit," he is overheard to mutter.

He squares up to her beside the bed.

"OK, Annie," he says. "I want you to stand." She does! "I want you to put your hands on my shoulders and pivot. We're going to waltz a little." Then he eases her onto the stretcher. By himself. A born leader of men. We were astounded. It generally took four firemen and two medics to accomplish what he had done with the voice of command alone.

Cutter used to be kind of a friend of mine. We thought in the same key. A colleague of ours quit his job to move back to his home state, because he heard that the unrequited love of his life had divorced. "That sounds like an excellent idea," I said. Only Cutter laughed.

After this, though, even after I tried to explain Annie's history to him, he decided I was a lazy malingering prima donna. I never really got along with him again. Cost me a job offer from his new service too. True, he himself had had a personality change. He used to be a funny, self-deprecating, pudgy, bustling short guy with a high level of competency and intelligence. He used the latter to become a humorless martinet, sprouting a bristly marine haircut, as supervisor. Rose in the profession, but his fatal flaw--a failure of empathy--kept him at risk in a volatile field. He had advanced in our service until one day when he failed to take a sexual harassment complaint seriously. He considered that bullshit too. It may well have been, but any supervisor who doesn't follow the sexual harassment protocol punctiliously is instantly out of a job. Another supervisor explained to me that if you ever get a second complaint, and you will, the lawyer easily uncovers that there was a "mishandled" previous complaint; so, since the company obviously didn't remediate the situation, it becomes pathetically liable.

Cutter was quoted to me as saying to the complainant, "Well, why don't you just give him a blow job and get it over with," but I think this is more firemen's humor. Cutter wasn't that stupid.

So what do we make of Big Annie? She definitely went to ground on purpose. She got something out of making nurses and medics and firemen struggle with her huge, half naked, smelly dead weight. What exactly did she get out of it? The cynical firemen maintained that she and her husband replayed, as foreplay, our struggles trying to lift her huge naked ass onto the stretcher.

"She likes the attention" is a kind of all-purpose formula for almost every psych patient, one that doesn't go very far. She also definitely called us for trivial reasons, like a possible sprained ankle. She was clearly more mobile than she let on.

At the same time, she probably did have maybe a year to live, and must have known this on some level. You can't be partially paralyzed, have had a stroke, be morbidly obese, be on 20 medications for assorted ancillary conditions, and expect to live long. But on the other hand, she hadn't given up. People are ambivalent. They have compartments. The left hand doesn't know the right. When I met her husband in the supermarket he told me about her diet. He certainly was in no way resigned to her departure. He was touchingly grateful for my efforts, physical and verbal. So Big Annie is a mystery. Which, actually, is one of the things I like about EMS. It's our fate to enter life in medias res, and depart before we hear the end of the story. It's our limited perspective that everything, even especially ourselves, can't really be fully explained.

So in my opening chapter about my first full arrest, if you can't figure out from what I said exactly where the firemen were, in front or in back of us, well, that's what a call is like, to say nothing of human memory. A serious EMS call is controlled chaos. You rigidly prioritize what you need to know and what you need to do, staying focused so the ghosts, wandering firemen, the wailing and gnashing of teeth in your peripheral vision don't distract you.

7 WILDERNESS

There was a box on my run form to indicate the environment of the call. The choices were rural, suburban, urban or wilderness. What I liked about my coverage area was the variety. SW Bexar county had old farms, some Hispanic and some German; it had growing suburbs, upscale and downscale; very old rural neighborhoods with porcupines and wild scenic properties, and some high rise business complexes and apartments which qualified as urban. The other thing I liked was that the local first responders were minimally trained. Instead of arriving on scene to find a paramedic fireman had already done everything, the whole intervention was my responsibility. I did all the work.

I really only took one honest to god wilderness call, though. Wilderness EMS is a thing apart. Medics learn extrication from ravines, high angle rescues, white water rescues, wild helicopter landings, transport on foot over rough terrain, a raft of boy scout lore.

We covered an army training base, many square miles of unimproved caliche roads, rocky hillsides and juniper brush, endangered species. About midnight we took a full arrest call there. We rendezvoused with a military team—took a while to find them—and set off through tunnels of scrub trees, bouncing over rutted dirt roads for miles, our progress lighted by lurid headlights shining into the juniper tunnels. It was awe inspiring only in a back of the mind kind of way, though, because our main concern was that you have less than ten minutes to intervene successfully in a full cardiac arrest. It took us more than 20 to come up on a knot of police and military standing around an obese sticky grimy corpse pulled half onto the caliche, dressed in by now filthy hunting togs. CPR was not in progress. It was merely a matter of recording an asystole flatline on two leads, checking for dependent lividity and pupillary responses. He was a deer hunter working a permit who had been found by someone hours or possibly even days after his fatal heart attack. I did get to check off wilderness on my run form.

I used to check it off at Sepulveda too, with arguable justification. This was a rural facility run by a Mrs. Sepulveda. She kept a collection of elderly schizophrenics and similarly handicapped folk in a rambling, leaning, L shaped building off I35 in a depressed rural area. You had to know where it was, since her I 35 address didn't match the entry, on a side street. In fact pretty much everything imaginable was dubious about the place. She called us more or less whenever an inmate became too bothersome for her, and shipped them to the worst hospital in town. They had kind of a symbiotic relationship, at least till the hospital realized she wouldn't take them back again. They always had to find other facilities. Being supremely inefficient, it took South Central literally years to figure this out and percolate it, but once they did, well, we spent one Sepulveda discharge transport hour driving all around town waiting for our Dispatch to find a destination for our patient.

In her back yard, Sepulveda had an above ground swimming pool and a trampoline. We used to imagine our elderly, hallucinating and handicapped patients diving into the pool or doing back flips on her trampoline as therapy.

Her patients universally accused her of stealing from them. Given most of them were clinically paranoid, and indigent, I tended to discount their stories, for a long time. Then it struck me as odd that every single one accused her.

She had a sidekick who handled most of the work, Mrs. S being rarely in evidence, except presumably when it came time to cash the Medicaid checks. Joe exasperated me at first since he seemed to know nothing at all about any of his patients and seemed to have no discernable medical training. You get used to arriving at a nursing home to find that the LVN can't give you a medical history on a critical patient she called you to help. "Well," she says, "we've only had him a couple days." We got a better history in our platinum ten minutes than she had managed in 78. She just couldn't be bothered. Nursing homes are desperately understaffed, so they can't fire people for sloth. The seven deadly sins just aren't what they used to be. Take gluttony, or pride. Avarice. And what's left of the periodical industry is based on envy.

Or we'd get a frantic call for respiratory distress with cyanosis. We'd show up to find the patient walking around, a "walkie talkie." She did have some age related discoloration on her heel. Same as under my boot, actually. During transport, we'd report these cases to the emergency room as "LVN panic" for chief complaint. Alternatively, you'd come for a routine transport to find a patient circling the drain, whom they had just noticed and then misdiagnosed as not serious. One nursing home noticed their ambulatory, talkative patient hadn't shown up for meals. So they went looking for him the next day and found him unconscious in his bed. Called us for "sick person." We took a call at a state psych facility for "unresponsive" to find an obese 34 year old black woman, indeed not responding. She had normal vitals, normal blood sugar, normal sinus rhythm and a psych history. She wasn't speaking or opening her eyes but her reflexes were intact. "Unresponsive" to us meant a Glasgow of 3: a patient with no reflexes, no pupillary responses and no speech: not responding. To LVN's it could mean dead, or alternately, someone who didn't feel like talking to them today. We brought the psych patient to the hospital. Didn't take a temp, since we had found her in a warm bed in a warm facility, and she didn't feel warm or cold. Had the transport been longer I would have gotten to it. It wasn't high on the list. Not like she was elderly. Turned out she was 94 degrees. Hypothermic. Our theory was: no one at the state hospital had checked on her for hours. Then they found her lying on the tiles on the bathroom. "Oh shit," they went, stuck her in bed, and called us. "We found her like that. Don't know her history, she's only been here a few days."

Joe, the sidekick at Sepulveda, also failed to inform us that his facility's rear door had a ramp. We had been carrying our stretcher up and down the front stairs for months before he mentioned it. I forgave him once I found out that, actually, he was a former inmate, with some cognitive deficits. He worked fulltime for Sepulveda, compensated by room and board, and her paying for some accreditation courses he needed to work there. He supported a son too. After finding that out, I was kind of a fan, and he became very fond of me. Didn't take much. "The other crew was really rude. I said, 'why can't you be nice, like that tall medic.'" To his further credit, I later found him on scene at a completely different group hell hole where he got a legitimate job doing the same thing. He still didn't know a thing, but he was still doing his best.

We did get some serious calls at Sepulveda, though even these were odd. Once we arrived to find a dwarf seizing. It's rare and very serious to arrive at a seizure call to find the patient still seizing, or seizing again, not faking. It's called status epilepticus and requires immediate oxygen, attention to the airway for vomit, IV access and valium to stop the seizure. People generally stop breathing during seizures. They can die. Usually you show up to find them post ictal--dopy and recovering. Cliff held down the poor little fellow's arm, I got a line in, shoved in the valium and he stopped seizing. He didn't regain consciousness, though, but his coma score was pretty high, and he had a good solid intact gag, so we let him snore rather than paralyzing him and intubating. Wilford Hall made the same choice, after we got him to the emergency room, so we felt vindicated. Big Willie is not shy about intubating. Still, he wasn't coming back. Cranial bleed? Some congenital condition? Dwarves are not normal, and Sepulveda dwarves had to be even more special.

So, at Sepulveda, we'd had to load him onto our stretcher for rapid transport. Usually Cliff and I worked together like a dance team, without a word spoken, but this time we got our wires crossed. I pulled when I was supposed to hold. The little guy nearly slipped into the crack between the bed and the stretcher, had not Cliff made an adroit save. Amazingly heavy for his size. Dense. Small legs and arms, all chunky. Heavy body.

"Stop larking about," I hissed at Cliff. "What do you think this is, a dwarf throwing contest?" He kept a straight face.

We took him to the adult side. Another medic once delivered a dwarf to pediatrics, and never really lived it down. We left him there, still snoring lustily.

"Well, something's not right," the doc said. "I guess we'll run some tests and try to figure it out." Yet another story without an end. Heisenberg didn't know the half of it.

We regularly got calls for assaults at Sepulveda. We were there for one thing or another at least once a month. Normally you stage for an assault, waiting nearby, but out of sight, for a sheriff's officer to clear the scene for safety. But we had long since relinquished our fantasy that Mrs. Sepulveda was being held hostage by armed freaks, a la Todd Browning. Anything she could handle, we could handle. So we'd cruise up without waiting for anything, often passing a staged fire truck. Intrepid medics.

I got to use Haldol the first time there. We had a combative patient who was, this time, a hale, chunky 30 year old woman with a deep grudge against Mrs. Sepulveda. She flatly refused transport. We stood over her, two big medics, a couple firemen and a sheriff's officer and told her she was going. She got the idea. As she was clearly a danger to others, having already assaulted Mrs. S, so we had every right to transport her by force if need be. She said she'd go if we let her walk to the stretcher. This struck everyone as reasonable. You empower people as much as you can. Leave them some autonomy and dignity.

However, it turned out her strategy was to suddenly dive at Mrs. S as she passed her in the doorway and land as many haymakers as she could before being pulled off by the sheriff's officer. Kind of a professional reflex, as no one really had any objection to Mrs. S taking a few healthy shots. So we ended up holding our patient down on the stretcher, exposing a vein and injecting a cocktail of Haldol and Versed, a fine time being had by all. It doesn't get any better. The Versed by itself had never been any use to us, we had to tie people down anyway, but this concoction turned her into a pussycat in minutes. A snoring pussycat in ten. I contemplated giving some to Mrs. Sepulveda, my favorite supervisor and the mean nurse at South Central too.

Most of the assaults, though, involved two long term patients called Harold and Floyd, a pair of elderly schizophrenics in poor health. It took us months to figure out the whole story. Harold had a small collection of plastic dinosaurs, about a foot long each. Whenever Floyd messed with his dinosaurs, there would be trouble. Fisticuffs. So when we cruised up one pleasant and sunny afternoon, this time by the pool and trampoline in the back, where the ramp was, I said, "So, Harold, what's up? Floyd been messing with your dinosaurs again?" The firemen, by now equally wise to Sepulveda, were already there. Harold was sulking and wouldn't answer. We called in another truck. We can easily take two noncritical patients on one transport, but given these two had been fighting, it didn't seem like a good idea to put them on a bench and stretcher less than a foot apart.

I assessed both Floyd and Harold. They were ambulatory, alert and in no apparent distress, normal vitals, warm, pink and dry, except Floyd had a bruised eye and Harold had a cut—lac—on his temple.

We had been toned out for an assault with possible head injury. Assault means no one is really hurt, but head injury is serious. I had found, though, that you had to be really tactful about what you wrote in the box for chief complaint. If you put chest pain, you had better follow the entire acute cardiac protocol, oxygen, IV, nitroglycerin, 12 lead EKG, aspirin. Or have an excellent reason for not doing it--patient allergic to aspirin or whatever. If the patient had a pain in his chest from an injury, or coughing, or straining a muscle, you had to be very careful to write "intercostal strain" or "rib tenderness" instead of CP, or you'd be in the station trying to explain to the wolves why you hadn't followed the chest pain protocol. And they would make you suffer anyway, not to be balked of their legitimate prey by mere common sense.

The same was true of black eyes and lacerations on the face. If the black eye resulted from a sufficient mechanism of injury, you'd call it a head injury, and put a cervical collar, back board and blocks on the patient to protect his cervical spine. But if it was 70 year old Harold flailing at 67 year old Floyd and grazing his eye, you were better off putting "eye contusion" or "facial laceration" in the box, without causing distress, struggling and possible injury by attempting to board the poor fellow.

The second medic arrived while I was still doing the assessment. He heard me asking both Harold and Floyd who was president. Harold said Truman, and Floyd said Nixon. Always ready to take the most dire case, as first medic on scene, I told the second medic, "I'll take Truman, you take Nixon." You have to realize that both gentlemen were psychotic, and this was their normal level of orientation. They were walking around and perfectly alert.

Pedro, the second medic, asked me if I thought he should backboard Nixon. "This is a head injury, right?" He was a punctilious, stickler type, who did not want to ask for trouble.

"Suit yourself, buddy," I said. "I'm not planning to board Truman. Good luck, by the way: Nixon fights restraints."

Pedro sniffed.

He elected for the full Monte. We transported 20 minutes before he did. En route to South Central, we heard Pedro initiate transport.

After a while, he got back on the radio to say he had been diverted by South Central to University, all the way on the other side of town. We were puzzled. We knew South was open, since they took us. Five minutes later his partner came back on the radio to tell dispatch they had been bumped up to code three, lights and sirens, by University. Had Nixon crashed? Had he fought the board and injured himself? Had a seizure? Many Sepulvedians had seizure disorders.

We found out at South Central that Pedro had called in the transport to South Central as a head injury. Well, South Central has no neurology, so they naturally declined. University was the nearest Level 1 trauma center (neuro), so Pedro diverted there. Then he'd called it in to University as a head injury again, and allowed that the patient had altered mental status, ALOC (altered level of consciousness). Which to be sure, being schizophrenic, he did. But it wasn't an ALTERED status, because he was normally like that. Well, naturally, University triage tore Pedro another one for even thinking about transporting a head injury with ALOC as a regular transport. So Pedro screamed into University, rushed his patient to the waiting assembled resuss team, and had a third one torn for him when the MD's found an alert though somewhat bewildered schizophrenic, no apparent distress, with a small laceration on his temple.

I did get to check the wilderness box though. Sepulvedaland.

I didn't check it for the guy with the avulsed scalp, though that was a messy rural call too. We arrived, hiking over some pastures, to find firemen mooning aimlessly over a 50 year old farmer who had run into an I beam on his tractor. He had succeeded in entirely skinning the right side of his scalp from his skull. Remarkably, he didn't seem to have knocked himself out—tough old German noggin—and an adult can't bleed out from his head, but he was still critical. He was ambulatory, so we attempted a standing take down onto our backboard. This WAS a head injury. The firemen didn't seem to get it, so our poor patient was teetering woozily while they were ineffectively aligning the board with his back. Making him squat down and crawl onto the board would've been totally stupid. The point was minimum manipulation of his spine. We finally got the maneuver accomplished, but I was seriously disgruntled. Not good patient care. You don't expect firemen to be medically competent, but they really ought to know how to use a backboard, especially since vehicle extrications are their job, not ours.

Then it pissed me off more to hear the thud thud thud of Air Life. The fire chief had launched. This patient was alert and oriented, and I had a 15 minute transport time to a level one trauma center, so Air Life was uncalled for. You use them if they can get a critical patient there at least five minutes before you can. Prolonged extrications, mass casualties. Serious I can handle myself. In fact, Air Life has never interested me as a job because they only handle trauma, don't see the whole scene, and, when there's a competent paramedic on the ground, they arrive to find everything has already been done for them.

New Braunfels Fire once responded to a motorcyclist who had the good fortune to wipe out right in front of an army medic truck in convoy. NB got there in three minutes, to be handed a slip of paper with the patient's vitals written on it, fully backboarded, c-collared, intubated, IV in place and ready to load.

Air Life had to assess my patient, load in a field, and unload at the helipad, so I could probably even have beaten them.

"Why did you call Air Life?" I asked the chief.

He shrugged. It was his call. He could see I was annoyed but he didn't want to get into a beef with someone he worked with every day, who was his superior, so he backed off. I could see he hadn't changed his mind, though, so I felt my competence being impugned. Then we got busy assisting

Airlife, giving report, transferring care and getting the patient on board, so I had a cooling off period. It's always engrossing to watch them launch.

The chief was one of the nicest people I knew. A volunteer too. He was an extraordinarily ugly dude, pockmarked and yellow snaggletooth, but he had a beautiful soul, easy to discern, shining through. His son worked in the department too and was equally estimable.

We were returning the stretcher and equipment to my rig when we walked by the accident scene, with the I beam slanting crazily up in the air.

"What was he doing anyway?' I asked mildly. I know nothing at all about farming but I'm curious about my district.

"Well," the chief said, considering. "Putting something up, I guess. Or taking it down."

I looked at him. We both grinned, perfectly aware that he had unwittingly summed up not just farming, but life as we know it.

8 FULL ARREST

The most glamorous calls, the ones every newbie fears and longs for, are the full cardiac arrest, and the really gory traumas, perhaps during a Mass Casualty Incident: defined technically merely as a call with more patients than medics, and governed in the texts by strict rules of triage. The moribund are abandoned to their fate (black tagged), the victims who can wait, wait (green), and your limited resources are poured into the critical who are most easily salvageable (red).

The trick in an MCI, actually, is not triage, but to find all the patients, who tend to be hidden, enter or leave the scene, be found in the wrong vehicle, or get themselves mixed up with bystanders, who, in turn, masquerade as victims.

The trick in trauma, no matter how dramatic, is to stop the bleeding, cervical collar and backboard, take vitals and transport as rapidly as possible. IV in route in a moving ambulance, call in report to the receiving facility, scramble to get as much done as possible Lots of fun. On rare occasions you may need to dart a chest to relieve pressure, or cut open a throat to insert a breathing tube into the cricoid membrane, but these will happen only once or twice in a career. The time I darted a chest during a traumatic arrest, blood came out, not air. It was a hemothorax creating the pressure, not a pneumothorax, and blood can't be effectively drained through a 12 gage IV needle, so it was pointless. Traumatic arrests are almost invariably unsalvageable anyway.

Medical calls are really more interesting. In theory paramedics aren't supposed to diagnose, but you have to figure out if an unconscious patient has had a seizure, or has low blood pressure, low blood sugar, an arrhythmia, or a stroke before you can help him, which can't always wait till the hospital. The most difficult differential, deciding between lungs and heart as etiologies, I finally just ran symptomatically, after not getting much help from even physicians in how to tell one from the other. Even in the hospital they're hard to tell apart, one told me. Plus they're usually linked anyway.

So the most interesting call cognitively, more rewarding ultimately than most full arrests, was congestive heart failure. CHF. You arrive to find Pickwick or Colonel Sanders, panting and often wheezing, sitting up, having already tried his nebulizer. He's usually obese, usually elderly, usually with a history of CHF or obstructive pulmonary disease or heart disease or hypertension or all of the above, but sometimes with recent onset, pale and clammy. His oxygen saturation is not good, and his carbon dioxide capnography worse. You hear burbly rhonchi in his chest. They sound like bowel sounds, but bowel sounds don't coordinate with breathing. You take a blood pressure. If it's over 100 systolic—and usually the patient will be hypertensive—you spray nitroglycerin in his mouth, after asking about his drug allergies, even if he is not experiencing chest pain. Then you get an IV. You put 40 mg of Lasix into the port. Lasix is a diuretic and will force his kidneys to pull fluid out of his body, i.e. lungs. He'll want to pee en route. Lasix works better after the nitro, and stresses the heart less, the nitro relaxing the vasculature and creating more vascular space, so the heart works less hard and has less blood pressure to fight. Also the heart itself is perfused better, the cardiac arteries being widened by nitro too. Then you nebulize the Colonel with albuterol, or albuterol and atrovent if he's maxed himself out already. Nebulize last. It can strain the heart but it also opens the lungs.

The Colonel's color improves. He breathes easier. You can chat about his service in World War Two. Get a wonderful story about Nijmegen.

If this all goes well you have the satisfaction of having shown some real gratitude for his service, far better than affixing a yellow sticker to your car, and also of having the doc at BAMC ask you "So what do you want me to do?" FIXED.

Hypoglycemic calls are good too. In our textbooks, diabetics have high blood sugars and are to be found in Diabetic Ketoacidosis, with fruity breath redolent of ketones, deep panting with Kussmaul breathing to vent acidity. But nowadays everyone is on insulin. So they overdose. We find them with blood sugars barely high enough to sustain life. Insulin shock. Usually they don't actually take too much insulin, they just forget to eat, or take Insulin anyway when they've been throwing up with flu or sweating in the garden.

One grampa liked to take his insulin, then walk next door to have breakfast with his daughter. He'd be loopy by the time she got it on the table, but he seemed to enjoy the high. Until she had to call us because he was too crazy to eat. He insisted on dancing with my partner. She's very good looking. You either talked him into eating-–it helped if you looked like my partner--or, if he went down, you wrestled with him, got IV access and shot an amp of D50 into him. Fixed. But then you must wait around to make sure he eats. The D50 wears off before the insulin. And if there wasn't a good explanation for why his sugar tanked, you'd transport. Or if he was too elderly and frail to object. The frail and elderly can't tolerate adventures like that well.

But the ultimate medical call is the full cardiac arrest. I ran about 25 during the five years I worked 911. It's sad I don't even remember most of them anymore, though my memory can still be jogged. That was a high incidence. I was a shit magnet when it came to full arrests, a white cloud as far as pediatric deaths. The luck of the draw, and I'll take it. I had six saves. A medic can go a whole 20 year career with just one or two, so I was both fortunate in the cases which came my way, and highly skilled. The constant practice helped immeasurably. You work faster, develop more adept and more accurate skills, and perform interventions more thoroughly, the more you practice. You have better clinical judgment and deeper medical knowledge. Having another skilled paramedic to assist helps a lot too.

I found one guy still sitting on his couch with a cigar still in his mouth. I was able to clear it, yank him to the floor, get firemen into CPR and ventilation, intubate and start an IV in the time it took the second medic to start one line. He was a good medic, too. Like an aerial dogfight, running a full arrest is a sport, kind of. Not quite as much fun as basketball, but on a higher plane, if you follow.

As for what a save is, the definition is not fixed. Physicians don't even use the word, I gather, but have a related concept. They talk about cases where they caught something serious, potentially lethal, which other docs had missed; or they employed an original treatment to the same end. By this standard I might have zero. It's hard to say, which may be why we don't use that rubric. Another medic on the same scene could have done just what I did, but the point is moot, because, unlike for the MD, there was no other medic. Cardiologists and ER docs use "save" to mean a cardiac arrest patient who walks out of the hospital afterwards. He's not permanently brain damaged or living on a vent. By that standard I had one full arrest save that I know. The others, again, I wouldn't know.

Our service defined "save" as finding a pulseless, apneic (not breathing) patient and getting him to the emergency room with a pulse and blood pressure, and then having that patient make it up to the intensive care unit. Again, contrived. Seems to rely on the emergency room too much.

On the street, a save is bringing a pulseless and apneic patient to an emergency room with a pulse (better, a normal sinus rhythm) and a normal blood pressure. Being a street medic, that's the standard I'm using. ROSC. Return Of Spontaneous Circulation. A simple miracle. Resurrecting a dead person. Dead by the ancient definition of no heartbeat.

My one indubitable case was a call for chest pain. He was a 41 year old darkly complected Hispanic seated on his couch in his neat suburban home attended by his wife. His main complaint, actually, was a terrible headache. His only history was a cerebral aneurysm that had been clipped. He was slender, no family history, no risk factors, didn't smoke or take stimulants. He was in good shape, muscular and trim. We initiated the acute cardiac protocol because he did indeed have chest pain, but I wasn't buying it. I was inclined to think his problem had something to do with the repaired aneurysm. In a male, the chest pain of an MI is usually pressure and usually radiates to the left arm or jaw, possibly middle of the back. Visceral nerves don't localize well and tend to group by spinal cord entry point rather than an organ system. Diaphoresis, profuse sweating, is my favorite indicator. Supposedly a sense of impending doom is common, but it's much more common in panic attacks, which can mimic myocardial infarctions pretty closely. This patient may have also had that typical greyish tinge, which I in this case I missed because of his dark complexion. So I thought it was his head, but we took a 12 lead EKG, started him on oxygen, gave him nitroglycerin and 320 mg of chewable baby aspirin, and started an intravenous line as per acute cardiac. I wasn't really happy about the nitro since it gives most people a headache. Seemed like increasing his intracranial pressure might not be a good idea. But his 12 lead was bad. In fact, with more experience, I would have recognized what we call tombstones: ST elevations which slant right up into peaked T waves. That is to say, his EKG indicated a localized injury to a specific part of his heart, such as would be caused by an occluded cardiac artery. This is called a STEMI, an ST Elevation Myocardial Infarct, which demands immediate notification of and transport to a cath lab for diagnosis and insertion of stents to hold open the occluded artery. Unfortunately, not everyone with a bad EKG is having a heart attack, and not everyone having a heart attack has a bad EKG. Unfortunately, I had just had a case where ST elevations meant nothing. That, however, had been a more elderly gentleman with a previous MI, who had just had stents inserted, so of course his heart showed as injured.

So our Chest Pain was not typical, but so far we had run everything according to Hoyle. Most MIs are not perfectly typical. We transported expeditiously. But not code three, lights and sirens. We were only 8 minutes from Wilford Hall even by regular transport so the difference would have been a minute or two. At that time we didn't notify cath labs in advance of arrival. I don't remember all of the call but I assume the patient was not actively feeling chest pain after our interventions. Otherwise I would have been running hot. Now I would anyway, because of the tombstones. Active chest pain and an abnormal EKG is a hot call. Active chest pain which is suspicious. STEMIs.

Still, everything was hunky dory. I was in back with the patient, still following the algorithm. Cliff was in front with the patient's wife. Then, not so good.

The patient slumped to his side, against the cabinets, shaking and no longer conscious. I figured his aneurysm, or another one, must have blown. I felt stunned. I looked at my monitor. It was showing V tach, a lethal rhythm typical of MIs. I yelled to Cliff to pull over and help. Everyone freaked, but in his own way. The wife froze and whimpered in fear, asking us what was happening. Cliff pulled over, set the lights, and ran around to the back, with his handheld radio. By the time he opened the back of the ambulance, I had pulled out the pediatric pacing pads from the monitor case, intending to paste them to my patient's chest to shock. I saw the little smiley faces, threw the pedi pads into the corner, and grabbed the adult ones. We were still getting used to this monitor, a fine new model. I put the pads on the patient, sternum and midaxillary, and checked my monitor again. The patient, unconscious and limp, was now in ventricular fibrillation, his heart quivering uselessly, which is the rhythm you shock V tach to prevent. I set the monitor on shock, set the joules at 200 biphasic, and then Cliff opened the back door.

"Stand clear, I'm going to shock," I said. I did.

The patient was fully restrained with shoulder straps and three sets of seatbelts, but he slammed into the cabinet wall, right up off the gurney. "Damn," I thought. I was impressed. I began chest compressions and Cliff climbed in, put the bag valve mask together, attached it to oxygen, put it over the patient's face and began to ventilate, once every five seconds. He called for backup on his radio.

We stopped after a minute and checked the rhythm. The patient was now in a wide complex very slow rhythm which is called agonal. Only the bottom half of his heart was working, and very slowly. Cliff continued compressions and ventilations and I got out the drugs I needed. I put a mg of epinephrine and then one of atropine into my IV line and ran it wide open. Patient had CPR pulses I could feel in his neck.

I tended to get stuck following the algorithm doggedly, so Cliff suggested another rhythm check. The patient's complexes were getting much tighter, more normal looking in shape, and much closer together. In fact, he was starting to look sinus, normal except slow.

After you shock, the heart stops. Asystole. Then it resets itself, but it takes a while to get both top and bottom working in a coordinated way. We felt for a pulse. All right! We took a blood pressure. By the time we got it, the patient was in a normal sinus rhythm. His blood pressure was adequate.

Cliff cancelled backup and went back up to the front to drive us to Wilford Hall. I could have hung an antiarrhythmic drip at this point, so the same thing wouldn't happen again, but we were two minutes from the ER and setting the drip takes time. Besides, the patient's rhythm looked terrific. He wasn't throwing any premature ventricular contractions, and his T wave electrical recovery was rapid and complete, so he didn't seem at immediate risk for another arrhythmia. His blood pressure continued to improve. I was just watching and keeping the oxygen flowing, after calling in the update to code three.

Pretty soon the patient's his eyes opened. He looked around.

"I got to pee," he said.

"I'm glad to hear it," I said.

A cloud passed over his face.

"What just happened?" he asked.

"Well," I said, considering how to answer. I never lie to a patient, but I also don't like to alarm someone in such a fragile state. More anxiety was not desirable. Basically, he had just died. I wasn't going to say that, though.

"Well," I said again, "you had a heart attack. You seem to be doing very well now though."

"Heart attack" didn't sound great, but I couldn't think of anything better. I considered explaining cath labs and blood tests for cardiac enzymes and the like, as I usually do with chest pain patients, but I was kind of exhausted, if also wired.

I decided to leave well enough alone. He probably wasn't ready to absorb a lot of medical information at the moment anyway. I don't remember what we talked about. He may have just lain there quietly, recuperating.

The docs were quite interested. The monitor automatically records shocks and rhythms so they were looking at the tape over each other's shoulders.

"So this is what you shocked," one said.

"Yeah," I said. It was pretty clearly ventricular fibrillation, so I didn't feel anxious about having done the wrong thing. I was kind of spaced, not tracking everything, and pleased. It turns out to be really easy to be a hero. Anyone can do it. You just need to be trained to use a cardiac monitor—an AED will do—and to be in the right place at the right time.

I was writing my run form when a nurse who had been in the trauma room when I reported walked by. The run form for a full arrest is voluminous. Cliff was outside putting our trashed ambulance back in order, figuring out what we needed to restock. A full arrest takes a while, but then you still have to go out on the next call right afterwards.

“So,” she said, “I guess this is what you did EMS for.’

“Yeah,” I said. “Sort of.”

It was kind of more complicated than that. Nurses know more than we do, and they do a wider range of things, but they do them in teams, and under a doctor’s direct orders. And they don’t intubate, spike chests, cut down throats for airways, or shock people. They don’t drive flaming screaming ambulances at high speeds. They don’t do rodeo sticks. They don’t run the call. We wouldn’t either, if we worked in a hospital. The US, however, doesn’t send MDs to people’s houses, lights and sirens. They send us. It works pretty well.

On the way out I passed the cubicle where my patient was in bed, sitting up next to his wife. He recognized me and gestured enthusiastically, wanting to thank me. I waved cheerfully. Now I would go over to get to know him a little, if not bask, but at the time I was feeling shy, perhaps coming down from the adrenalin.

My high school dance and deportment class hadn’t covered this situation. Learning the Lindy was simple enough given enough time, but it had seemed overwhelmingly complicated to introduce your partner to the hostess. Crossing over behind her and what not. Frozen with fear, I’d resolved to just mimic the guy in front of me, Mark Landis. So I shook hands with the host, looked the gentleman in the eye, and said, “Good evening, I’m Mark Landis.” Fortunately I said it so softly that he didn’t notice, not being that interested anyway.

What to say to someone who’s thanking you for saving his life hadn’t come up.

I remember doing one with another paramedic who was a volunteer in the fire department, but also worked as a medic for Austin, the best service around. I got the tube and he got the IV; then he earnestly and industriously injected not only vasoconstrictors but also antiarrhythmic, and finally set a dopamine drip for blood pressure, and an antiarrhythmic drip.

Wilford Hall was impressed. I'd set similar drips myself, but he'd done a very good job.

The dopamine was too fast, though, making the patient tachycardic. Once I'd transferred care I couldn't really reset it, and the MD assumed mine was working. Only a nurse was unhappy.

"Aw, a little tach won't hurt him, after a full arrest," the doc said.

"Well the dopamine's all gone now anyway," she muttered bitterly, after a while.

The patient did as well as could be expected. Making some attempts to breathe when we left, but still deeply unconscious.

I arrived in the narrow back bedroom of a beat up old house ten minutes (I clocked it) after the first crew. The paramedic was still trying to intubate. I took over, dropped the tube (the patient was an easy tube), moved to her arm and set an IV. The paramedic had drilled an intra-osseous (IO) into her tibia without even trying for an IV. Supposedly an IO works as well as a line, but it doesn't. It's slow, for one thing. We ran in all the drugs for an asystole arrest. During a rhythm check we saw a slow sinus. I felt her carotid. "I've got a pulse," I said. The woman's friend, hovering anxiously by the bed, said "Oh thank God." None of us said anything. The patient had blown pupils—I'd checked—indicating severe brain deterioration, so I wasn't sanguine. The eyes are called the window of the soul in poetry. In EMS the pupillary response—cranial nerves go directly to the brain without passing through the spinal cord—give us a snapshot of what's happening inside the bone walls of the skull. Pupils which are fixed and dilated, soon aren't even round. They say no one's home. The soul has fled. Been down too long. We boarded and collared the patient. The medic's really powerful 270 lb. partner had the strength to tip the board up enough to lever it out of the narrow bedroom. A save, under the meaning of the act, but one I'm sure didn't walk out of the hospital.

"How many IOs have you done?" I asked the medic.

"I've already put in eight this year."

She just holstered the drill on her hip and pulled and fired at will, apparently. I'd done three in two years. If you can't get IV access, it's a lifesaver. Though one RN in an ER asked me to take it out again, the patient not needing it any more. "Sorry," I said, "we only know how to put them in." He looked sourly at the patient's leg. I mean, it's a surgical procedure.

When I told an orthopedist about them, he said, "Oh, I guess you just rough dissect the skin—but what do you do about the saphenous vein and nerve?"

"The what?" I said.

We just drill right into the flat spot below the knee, like putting a screw into a stud, pull out the bit, aspirate the cannula for blood with a syringe, and attach the IV catheter, flush and go. Only in life threatening emergencies.

I told our on duty supervisor about the call, on the quiet. He was a good friend of mine. Nothing happened. He knew how to keep himself out of trouble. Follow the rules and don't make waves. The constant turnover at my service, and the propensity of brand new medics to elect to work in the county, on 911 trucks, for the experience and glamour, despite the lower pay and terrible hours, meant that a lot of inexperienced crews were menacing the county at any given time. HQ was clueless about a lot of things, including how to keep good medics and fire bad ones.

We climbed a narrow stair to a bedroom where an 85 year old--but hale, white maned and chest haired--male was spiraling down into bradycardia, his heart beating slower and slower, losing a palpable pulse. I stuck the pacing pads on him and we stabilized his heartbeat temporarily with external electrical pacing. Since the stair was so narrow, two strapping firemen had to carry him down on the backboard, one in front, one in back, with the monitor balanced on his thighs. I'd impressed upon them fervently not to dump the monitor.

They succeeded, quite a feat of strength and coordination. But then, in the living room, kind of standing down, mission accomplished, they dislodged the monitor while heaving him onto the stretcher. It crashed to the floor. Bless its durable, conscientious heart, it continued to pace, undeterred. Even the lines were long enough to hold. We brought him back alive.

I did one with Bruce Ritchie which was pretty interesting too. I was first medic so I was getting the IV when he walked in. I asked him to tube. He'd been my field training officer but by then I had more recent practice than he did and was more current on the drugs and protocols. We were both pretty confident. The more calls you run, the more used to the drill you become. We put in antiarrhythmics, vasopressors, a pharmacological cornucopia. I was sitting by the patient's IV arm counseling our student about what to draw up and how to calculate the dosages.

There's a clock method which works well because the drip set is 60 drops a minute. It took me a while to figure out WHY it worked though. I was anticipating coming into an ER and having the doc ask me why I had set the drip at the rate I did. "Well," I would say, "the big hand was on the...."

By now I had it down, though. We used only two drugs as drips, so I couldn't see why any medic shouldn't be proficient with them before having to use them, math and science fear or not.

Bruce was sitting by the head end near his tube. The student was standing by the mantelpiece with the drug box, holding up the running IV bag. Kind of a pajama party, a group of old trusted friends sitting around on the floor engrossed in a particularly challenging parlor game.

I was very fond of Bruce even without the male bonding kicking in. He was supremely equable, and just had a deep interest in other people. Many medics are cool under pressure but with him it didn't even look like he was controlling himself. He'd just look around brightly, enjoying himself, even once when I had dropped an essential part of a mechanical ventilator underneath a patient who was dependent on it to breathe. Bruce had calmly reached over and attached him to another device while I was fruitlessly diving under the stretcher for the dropped valve.

This patient was a fifty year old male, a witnessed arrest, with CPR started immediately, and our truck there within 8 minutes. All the same, he presented in asystole, flatline, so even after trying everything for 30 minutes, there was no return of spontaneous circulation.

Bruce and I were ready to pronounce, but the family wanted us to transport. We would do that as a matter of courtesy. If they imagined the hospital could do something an hour late which we hadn't already done, let them feel everything had been tried.

At 35 minutes, though, ROSC! Return of spontaneous circulation. We boarded, blocked and cervical-collared the patient to keep Bruce's tube in place. As we were loading, the drug box fell out of the basic's hands and scattered its contents all over the driveway. We left him to clean it up. We had my drug box in my ambulance, untouched.

So Bruce and I were sitting there in the back. "Did you see the drug box?" he said. He always thought I was unobservant but, though I look blind, probably from inner concentration withdrawing the life from my eyes, I really don't miss much. "Yeah," I said. "there's always something." Controlled chaos.

The drips had been set, the blood sugar checked, the bicarbonate for alkalinity infused, the patient in a sinus rhythm with a normal blood pressure. A fireman was still bagging him--breathing through Bruce's tube for him with the bag valve mask—and he was still unconscious. Pupillary responses were minimal. Not much brain function.

Bruce and I looked at each other. He was the most cheerful medic I ever met. Good humored and patient. Tremendous skills.

He'd come on a scene once with ET tubes littering the ground. "I guess you had trouble tubing," he said to the fireman. He picked up a tube, wiped it on his EMT pants and inserted it.

"Really?" I said, "What size blade did you use?" I liked the curved Mac 3 myself.

"Whatever was handy," he said.

Now, "can you think of anything else we can do?" he said over the siren. He was happy. This was only his second save in an 18 year career. Techniques and meds had improved and I was up on all of them by then.

"Well," I said, "we could do a 12 lead and see what caused this."

Bruce swiftly attached the 12 lead EKG, ran a strip, and, sure enough, ST elevations in leads 2 and 3. Tombstones. An occlusion of the LAD artery, called the widowmaker, which feeds the septum of the heart and the main ventricle. That accounted for the arrhythmia, as the septum controls pacing.

An MI, myocardial infarction.

We were still running hot to the nearest hospital as per protocol.

"Maybe we should bypass and head right for a cath lab," I said.

"Yeah," Bruce said, considering. "His chief complaint is coronary artery occlusion. We can bypass South Central." Which did not have a cath lab to run a catheter up from the patient's groin to the artery and open it up.

Bypass "the nearest facility." Divert OURSELVES. Aggressive and interesting.

Neither of us was really comfortable with it though.

"Nah," I said. "I think his chief complaint is death. I think we better stick to South Central."

The nearest appropriate facility. Unless it's on diversion, owing to too many patients. Then you find another hospital, or you have the authority to open them up. I've spent 20 minutes calling and cruising around looking for a facility.

Puts you in a ferocious mood. ERs clogged with people with no health insurance, using them as walk in clinics.

The MD on duty at South Central was a tall slender African I was very taken with. He seemed very intelligent and genteel. He had an air of reserve, dignity and quiet confidence. His way of giving you his full attention while visibly holding back emotionally was caressing in a respectful way.

He was not all that happy to see us and the subject of a cath lab never came up. The family had followed us to the hospital and arrived suspiciously close on our rig. They hadn't been following us with their flashers on like some suicidal idiots. We'd warn them not to do that.

The doc told them the prognosis was very poor.

"The paramedics did an excellent job," he said, "but he's been down too long."

His point of view was that it might have been better if we hadn't achieved a "save." This patient had a chance, but only at life in the ICU, on a vent, feeding tube and pressors. His chance of returning to consciousness was nil.

And this is why the nonperfusing rhythm algorithms stop after 30 minutes. We were ready to pronounce at that point, and then agreed to transport only as a courtesy to the family. By a long shot we achieved ROSC. Return of spontaneous circulation. The magic acronym. You bring him back from the dead. But that does not mean you're going to like what you bring back. Particularly with sick, frail, elderly patients. I mean, just think. They're not going to be in better shape than before they arrested, after you've smashed their chests and dosed them with powerful drugs, shocked their hearts. Usually, fortunately, you don't get anything back. So the cath lab was out. Yes, our patient could be transported to one, to have his heart fixed, as it were, and made strong enough to power a vegetable existence indefinitely.

You've gathered by now that the perspective of a paramedic is not the same as a layperson's. Nowadays, readers, the few that are left, seem to want inspiration, something that makes them feel good. Or why read? But it will come as no surprise to an adult, that teachers, speaking among themselves, doctors, policemen, tend to have a much darker vision of their clientele and profession than they would communicate in a funerary or celebratory speech.

There's a case to made against iconoclasm. You don't want to scare or discourage people or make them cynical.

But my vote is for realism. I highly recommend the scientific method. It should ideally inspire readers to consider their eating habits and life style, their votes concerning health care, their decisions about their own and their families' medical care. It's better to have a heart attack late in life in a hospital bed, rather than early in an ambulance, but the best is not to have one at all.

9 HISTORY

I was frozen with fear in my EMT class. I used to take a big fleece with me and wrap myself in it while everyone else was in T shirts. I hadn't been in a class in 25 years, and this new profession had no relation to my old one, which had fizzled out. For a while I was a house husband, but by now the kids were in school most of the day. A lot of my family were in medicine, it was shortly after 9/11, so, and, well, this may surprise you, but there are amazingly few interesting medical specialties which can be practiced with just a year of training. EMT Basic was two and a half months--two evenings and Saturday every week--then another few months for Intermediate, and only about a year total for Paramedic. I went straight through, though EMS people advise practicing a year at each level. MDs and RN's go straight through, I figured, and paramedic is the fun part. I didn't want someone else to be in charge—I tend to have problems with authority--or people yelling at me because I got lost on the way to a hospital, or messed up on the radio. I mean, I held the mike backside up for a while. My focus was medicine, patient care.

The class was a motley crew. A felon, who discovered he had to drop out, a mortgage broker losing his referrals, a waiter, a clothing store salesperson, two med school dropouts, an anesthesia tech, the single mother of a severely disadvantaged child, who advertised in class that her mother had taught her how to suppress her gag reflex.

I figured the mortgage broker, who was extremely intelligent, loud, obscene, an unorthodox thinker and practical joker, and his Anglo ally, a 19 year old woman, a 6 ft. heavy set fabulist, also loud and dramatic, would provide the center of gravity. He brought his boombox to the final exam, turned it on full blast to salsa, and then said, when everyone glared, "Hey, it relaxes me!" before turning it off. He had been divorced by a drug abusing nurse who had left him with an 8 yr. old son she inherited from a previous husband, taking the three houses he was using as rental properties. So he would only describe his present commonlaw, with whom he had his own child, as his girlfriend, so she couldn't do likewise. Naturally, she also left, leaving him doubly bereft.

The fabulist claimed to have sung at Carnegie Hall, to have inherited a house from strangers, and to drive a gold, loaded PT Cruiser no one ever saw. She boasted of having won a local amateur strip contest in the heavy breast category, stripping out of her fireman's uniform. Years later I saw her on the news, claiming to have been abducted.

The volunteer fire department she worked for inherited a house to burn for practice. She was upstairs with the hose when another volunteer noticed the attachment to the hydrant wasn't to his liking. He unscrewed the hose. She was hanging out the window, flames behind her, yelling they had no water. The fire chief traced and discovered the problem. He coldcocked the volunteer. THEN he reattached the hose.

However, four Hispanic males--the waiter, the salesman and two cohorts—effortlessly ran the class. The salesman was the leader. A genuinely suave character, he had a huge amount of quiet charm, much of which consisted of a perspicacious, profound interest in people. He noticed or divined everything about you, and appreciated it.

Only two other people besides me made it straight through, the anesthesia tech and one of the ex med students. I was always a good student. I did have to read and underline each chapter four times, even before studying for the National Registry exam.

A lot of warm feelings and camaraderie. The beginning of the "watch your back" ethos. I'm still fond of most of them.

The difference between handling a text and a patient, is, you must know everything about the artwork, in depth, and then you make an original interpretation. The patient you know hardly anything about, only what you can gather in ten platinum minutes. And your treatment better not be original. Apply the appropriate protocols.

We trained in hospitals, learning to listen to lungs, start IV"s, NG tubes, do physical exams. We rode out on ambulances as students. The medics mostly just let you follow them around, but sometimes they would let you try some interventions, or take a history and physical. I'm the only medic I ever met who would actually teach my students anything about the medical conditions they encountered. I enjoyed it.

I remember my student patients better than I remember the one I had an hour ago.

I got so little time in hospitals, due to proctors failing to show, that I learned to stick on the box: do IVs in my truck. So, like the Sundance Kid, I shoot better when I move. Conversely, in hospitals there are many true artists with a needle who can hit stationary veins I can't even see or palp.

You ride in the back as a student, so most of the time you don't know where you are or what's going on. We were on our way back from a call once when suddenly the rig lit up, started to howl and accelerated through a U turn. We screamed a few miles and stopped. The medics hopped out. I was disentangling myself from the seatbelt when the side door popped open. A fireman in turn-out gear said,

"Watch your step, buddy. There are brains all over the road."

I gingerly skirted small fluffy pink piles of what looked a bit like cotton candy.

Brains stink. Immediately.

A poorly dressed 30ish man lay supine on the pavement, the back of his head crushed and flattened into the asphalt. His head was tipped up into sniffing position. Perhaps someone had started to intubate. He'd been clocked crossing the road by an SUV driven by an off duty policeman vacationing with his family. It struck me that, given the fire crews, police, medics and Airlife (cancelled), this was probably the most money that had ever been spent on him in his life. Maybe some medical insurance or psych meds or drug rehab or housing or job training at an earlier point would have been more useful.

The lead medic was mad because a firemen led the off duty officer past the body. His SUV had a head shaped depression in the windshield. A human body is big enough to total a car.

You worry about a lot of things when you are starting out. Will you be able to handle the stress? Will you be able to stay calm, not freak out or freeze, and remember and perform the right exams and interventions rapidly and efficiently? Will the smells make you nauseous, the sights queasy? Will you save someone's life or will you kill someone?

I came home really late, showered the blood and sweat off me, and went to sleep. In the middle of the night I woke up nauseous, flashing back to the smell of brains. "Oh, shit," I thought. I had seemed to be handling it all right on scene. .

It turned out, though, that I had fortuitously contracted stomach flu.

As it turned out, I could stay calm and focused, and remember the protocols under stress. Inexperienced basics or firemen would criticize me—not to my face--for being too slow or too calm, until they were shown my on scene times. The trick with any movement sport, basketball or EMS calls, is not agitation but efficiency, not warmth and compassion but ice cold calm. Oscar Robertson usually looked like he was cruising.

Until you realized he had a step on his opponent. The Big O. Oprah is nothing.

Not that I was calm, especially in the beginning. I just looked calm. If everything was going well, I'd be quietly exhilarated. If not, I'd be on the edge of panic inside. But I kept my face calm and my voice low, soft and lazy, the way it usually is. It's a mild speech impediment, actually. Has a name I forget.

The best medics didn't even look calm. They looked like they were quietly enjoying a cocktail party.

In the beginning, medics are frightened. They have trouble handling complex calls. There's a lot to learn all at once. The radio, the truck, the equipment, the medicine. But it's all quite finite finally, unlike being a physician. We have a limited number of drugs, a small set of tools. So then medics settle in and enjoy themselves. Finally, many become cynical and torpid.

I'm kind of remote and interior. I probably don't fully engage during many human interactions. I tend to feel indifferent, not fully there. Stress may just wake me up to an average level of arousal. I used to enjoy final exams, SAT's, and dislike games. The exams were games that had a purpose.

But many types of people make good medics. More don't. The professional secret is that the normal response to a person collapsing or mangled, of "God, what do I do?" and the mixture of fear and horror, the clashing desires to escape and to help, but not knowing how, changes with professional training and experience. You feel, if not comfort then at least habituation, and you know perfectly well what to do. Plus you're not alone. Fire crews, experienced partners, you ride their shoulders even when you're in charge.

It's a deep source of satisfaction to know what to do. I'd like to see everyone take EMT Basic in high school. Leave out the equipment training, radio and truck expertise, but teach everyone some basic physiology and anatomy, not least so they can manage their own and families' health, and show them what to do in standard emergencies like bleeding, passing out, trauma, cardiac arrest.

It would be hard to teach people how to manage emergencies, though. There's a character and personality dimension, but experience is the best teacher. Knowing you can cope is a sense of solid ground under your feet. The sense there's a tungsten steel milled gyroscope residing in your solar plexus, ticking over quietly until it's needed. Your interior face takes on that expression common to large predators, like wolves and lions at rest, surveying the forest with a calm generated by their sense that there's nothing in there they can't handle.

I weathered the stress, the bodily fluids, the smells, the sights just fine. Or as fine as can be expected. Until I didn't. But that's a story for another chapter.

10 SMELLS

Every medic has a bodily fluid they don't like. It can't be blood. The blood of strangers is our livelihood. Everyone loves blood. It's such an amazing color, to start with. Such an amazing substance, too, the clotting, the homeostasis, the oxygen capacity, the immune devices. So powerful, so fragile. It fixes everything, and people are tough, but within minutes of exposure or stopping circulation it becomes a gooey poison. When patients tell me they could never do what I do because they faint when they see blood, or are scared of needles, or they tell me they've never been in an ambulance before, I have a stock response. "Isn't that a coincidence?" I say, "me too!" They look at me suspiciously for a minute and then smile.

Cliff loved snakes, was afraid of spiders and hated snot and phlegm. Plenty of medics dread abdominal bleeds, not so much the deadly low blood pressure, but the sticky, coffee-ground diarrhea, or the vomited feces emulsed with coagulated blood, the staggering reek. Blood becomes jello when there's enough of it. It disaggregates into red and yellow and white sections like a lethal pudding.

I have hardly any sense of smell any more, I've always had a strong stomach, and I find you screen out every distraction when you're working hard in extremis, so I could afford to laugh at the fireman who started to gag while he was doing chest compressions. We were on our knees in the patient's vomit, diarrhea and urine, sure enough. The fireman had to go outside and retch, much to all the crews' amusement. Time goes so quickly when you're having fun.

The one call which did make me queasy involved my least favorite fluid, which is stale, old lady urine. And yes it does smell different than old men's. This woman was about 65. Her housemate, to whom she'd rented a room, had called 911 when he noticed, after he came home, that she had not left her recliner.

Not for four days, it turned out. The old recliner hadn't smelled good even before she had used it as a toilet for most of a week. Her kidneys were one organ system which was working quite well. Furthermore, she had four cats. The nasal evidence indicated that they had come to the conclusion that if their mistress could let fly anywhere she felt like, so could they. Cat urine is seriously pungent, ammoniated.

We lifted her onto our stretcher, using her sopping nightie as a draw sheet. We covered her as best we could with sheets and blankets. It wasn't enough.

My partner offered to take the call. It just goes to show that there's good and bad in everyone, because I consider her to be the worst partner I ever had, and I had some doozies. One was determined to get me fired so she could move a friend into my spot. She wrote me up every day. Fortunately, the person who read the complaints knew me quite well and had enough savvy to read between the lines. It was still a big problem.

This particular partner, though, used to stand between me and the patient, and try to do my job instead of hers. She was supposed to get a blood pressure, collect meds and documents, while I took the history and did the exam, but she incorrigibly reversed roles. She may have wanted to be a paramedic, but I did not want to be a Basic, and I did not trust her abilities. She would yell at patients, take shortcuts, practice above her scope, and she had terrible clinical judgment. She'd be scrupulously washing the blood off a man's face who had just been knocked unconscious and had seized, instead of getting in front and driving me rapidly to the hospital while I did more crucial interventions. She counseled a guy with a pulmonary embolism to slow his breathing down as though he were having a panic attack. She was quite surprised when he died, though I had seen he was circling the drain from first sight.

But in this case she was bustling around in the back of the ambulance, turning on all the blowers and vents, keeping herself moving to calm her stomach. No one is all bad. Even Hitler liked dogs.

At the transport agency I worked for later, one of the medics posted a scrupulous imitation of the official notices entitled, "Fat Free Friday." It read, "Starting next month, Grim Reaper Ambulance [not its real name] will be instituting Fat Free Fridays. If you should encounter a patient who is more than a hundred pounds overweight, inform him or her, politely but firmly, that GR Ambulance will not be able to transport him or her till Saturday." A few medics bought it, management was furious, and the rest of us thought it was funny.

"How about No Stink Thursday?" one said. A female medic, whose patient had exposed himself to her that week, said, "No Wiener Wednesday." She hadn't had bodily fluid thrown at her a la Silence of the Lambs, like my other partner.

Patients have suppurating wounds, diarrhea infected with C diff, which you can diagnose from the hallway, gangrenous decubitus wounds. The sick don't smell so good. And hospitals don't seem to clean their patients anymore. Understaffing, I suppose. Despite 10% unemployment and royal medical reimbursements. It used to be every patient got a bath every day. Now hospitals are concerned about epidemic C diff, MRSA and other hospital borne infections which complicate care and even kill people. Seems like washing would be a start.

As for the obesity epidemic, that's worth a chapter of its own, if not book or two.

As for Cliff and the snakes and spiders, he once flatly refused to enter a house with a giant web over the door, and, during our snake bite call, while I was ministering to the patient in the back of the truck, he disappeared, totally unlike him. We always know where our partner is, like Siamese twins. I'd bandaged her up and called it in to Wilford Hall Medical Center by the time he showed up with a plastic bag. We don't do much for snake bites. Keep the affected part level with the heart and support blood pressure, monitor for arrhythmias. But in theory we can bring the snake so the hospital can determine what kind it is. Not that there will be much doubt in Texas. There are four poisonous varieties and everyone can tell one from the next. But I let Big Willie know we were going the extra mile.

"Do Not, repeat Do Not, don't you bring a live snake in here," the doc said. "Negative, do you hear me? No live snakes."

"Yes sir. It'll hurt my partner's feelings, but received."

It broke Cliff's heart to have to kill the poor little thing. "Aw, it's only a little guy." He'd been to a lot of trouble trapping it with a shovel against an interior door and bagging it up. The docs at Wilford Hall were as fascinated as anyone else. Could barely get them to attend to the patient.

Still, "if you'd brought it in here alive," one told my partner, "it'd be you I was intubating."

Don't cut into the bite, don't tourniquet, don't suck out the venom, and only 6 people per year die of indigenous snake bites. Nasty wounds though. Anti-venin is a last resort. Snakes don't even inject half the time. And anti-venin goes in with lots of Benadryl since very few people can tolerate IV horse serum. That's what anti venin is made of.

11 THE PROFESSION

EMT speech is quite formulaic. They're not writers. The culture is pre literate, with Homeric formulae rolled smooth and perfect like pebbles in a brook. There are black sheep and white clouds, BS calls ("another life saved"), radio traffic (sometimes "unreadable"), saves and bad calls, patient reports and patient info (not the same: do not mix up), the usual paramilitary acronyms and abbreviations: some of it medical speech.

EMS is said to stand for "Earn Money Sleeping," and it is true that medics, like off duty predators, sleep as much as they can, partly because of the long hours. Most stations run on 24/48 shifts. You're on for 24 hours and then off for 48, 365 days a year, with perhaps a two week vacation, which many medics cash in instead of taking. On top of that, many medics work extra shifts on their days off. The hourly pay rate is so modest that a medic can only make a decent wage by racking up overtime. You see them in the station or posted under an overpass or in a convenience store or lying on the unit's bench or draped on the front seats with the diesel running, snoring lustily. They have the uncanny ability to sleep through all the radio traffic, but wake up instantly when their unit number is called, even though they may be working a different shift with a different number.

They're close to firemen, of course; in fact many of us are firemen, but also akin to cops. We wave when we pass each other's units. Further, when you run into a cop when you're in uniform, he actually looks at you, speaks to you and generally interacts with you as if you were a person like himself, which he certainly does not do with "citizens," whom he does not trust. He doesn't regard citizens as the enemy exactly, though he knows they can get him in trouble, but more as potentially dangerous livestock he must shepherd. Whereas felons are colleagues, in a way, though also despicable.

We get a lot of respect generally, but cops' is the most gratifying. Law enforcement isn't a high status profession, but people do surmise the service and heroism. I worked in a state where uniforms are valued.

The reason firemen work as medics is simple. First, EMS is the youngest of the three professions, the Cinderella, and so gets the worst deal in wages, benefits and job security. The age of unions and public works had passed by the 50's and 60's and 70's when EMS was being organized in response to the epidemic of trauma, mostly vehicular. Then, firemen became more and more expensive and did less and less. Their equipment kept becoming more sophisticated and of course nothing is standardized in the US, and at the same time fires became fewer as housing construction, clothing, heating apparatus, fire alarms and sprinkler systems continued to improve. People smoked less. So a goodly number of these expensive gentlemen could be found sitting around, sometimes for days, doing very little, other than sleeping, though of course ready for anything. Hey, someone said, why not let them respond to the EMS calls too. They do anyway as first responders or to help with traffic control, vehicle extrications and fire suppression during motor vehicle accidents, so why not perform the medical care too? So dual function fire departments take EMS calls 80%, fire 20%. Depressing if you like fire but hate medicine, scary if you like EMS but don't care for running into burning buildings. But there it is. Earn money sleeping.

Transport agencies employ medics who carry patients from one facility to another. Nursing home residents to their appointments or to the hospital, surgical patients to follow up care, the bedbound to dialysis. To some extent they become ambulance drivers, but these patients are being transported in an ambulance for a reason. They crash. When they do, the first impulse is to say, "Jesus Christ! Someone call 911!" Then you realize that's you.

A bit like when you start out in the field, after your classes are passed. The shock is, they actually expect you to do all the stuff you practiced on the plastic dolls. I mean, for real. And, like, constantly, not just in a, well, emergency.

911 services don't work for the facilities, they work for the patients. So where the transport medic has to be extremely politic with even the most incompetent LVNs or facility coordinators—they're his bread and butter—and tread careful lines between making his own medical decisions and following handed down orders from MDs who may not even have seen the patient, 911 paramedics are required to seize control of a scene, put the patient first, and brush aside anyone who gets in the way, having him removed in cuffs by law enforcement if necessary.

If there's a complaint, the director checks it out. He's well connected, knows the mayor and the chief of police. If he decides the medic was right, he tells the complainant. What's he going to do, call another 911? Whereas the client of a transport service will do just that.

Being soft spoken and not bred to the profession, there was some concern in the beginning about whether I could be aggressive enough. It was unfounded. I can be as unpleasant and overbearing as the next person, and there's a chain of command which every paramilitary professional understands quite well. Half of them are ex-military. Insubordination is rare, and close to never if the subordinates judge you're making the right moves.

Everyone's first Strobos anecdote occurred quite early in my tenure, after I took over a position at a busy 911 post. In fact, I took over the position of my last field training officer. It so happened he wore the same size pants as I do, and he left a couple pairs behind. I asked if he wanted them back, but he had ordered new ones by then. I ran into him a couple weeks later and he asked how things were going.

"Well," I said. "I don't know if I'm filling your shoes, but I am wearing your pants."

Anyway, back to the anecdote. We responded to an elderly gentlemen with COPD (chronic obstructive pulmonary disease) who was having trouble breathing. His oxygen SATs were low, he was wheezing and laboring to breathe, and a stethoscope established he wasn't moving a lot of air. We put him on a nonrebreather mask with 100% oxygen at 12 liters a minute and began nebulizing. This stabilized his condition, without fixing it, but I still found the blood coming out of his nose alarming. There are a number of very serious lung complications which involve breathing out bloody froth. I elected to run him code three (lights and sirens, emergent) to the nearest facility, which was also a level one trauma hospital.

What I took to be a first responder emerged from the chaos of bystanders, family and neighbors, crews, to insist the patient had a right to choose his hospital. This faux responder had on the same color T shirt and the same kind of pants as the NW fire crew on scene with me, many of them new to me. I was enraged. To be sure the patient does have that right, but fire crew attempting to check mate my plan of action?

"You," I said, "off scene!"

Unfortunately, it transpired, the gentleman was the patient's son. While we were moving, I was busy stroking and apologizing, explaining that I was worried about his father and felt he should go emergent to the nearest hospital. He was mollified.

It turned out the patient was an ordinary COPD exacerbation with a fortuitous nosebleed but, despite ragging from the ER techs, I stand by the decision. Unless I knew for certain it was a nosebleed, why would I take the risk?

Nevertheless the incident was much discussed back at HQ and among the crews. EMS is a small, gossipy world. My On Duty Supervisors thought it was funny but they were indulgently approving. "He tried to throw the patient's son off scene! Thought he was a NW fireman!" The underlying tone below the ribbing was approval. They were reassured I was being aggressive, able to seize control of a scene.

Volunteer fireman are wonderful people, but also riff raff. Country. The medic on the shift after me, who knew all of them well, asked me how I had come to make this misidentification.

"Well," I said, "he was wearing a navy blue T shirt and he had on dark blue cargo pants, too, cpo's."

"Well," Keith said, "but did he have any teeth?"

"Teeth? Well, yeah—I mean, what do you mean, did he have any teeth?"

"Well," said Keith, laughing, "you ought to have known if he had any teeth he couldn't be a NW fireman."

NW fire people were always hiding their personal trucks at our station to keep them away from repo crews, or absconding with county funds.

Moose used to tell stories about being rejected on internet dates because he paid everything in cash out of a roll from his pocket, never realizing why that seemed ominous. He was great cook, though, and used to feed us Thanksgiving and Christmas dinners when we were on shift those days. We were grateful, and well fed.

He and his brother disappeared, but not before he'd responded to a multiple motor vehicle where we had to call San Antonio Fire for backup, as we didn't have enough crews available.

The SAFD medic was standing by the crumpled door of a sedan with two victims trapped inside when Moose walked up.

"Get the jaws," the medic said.

"You mean you want the door open," said Moose

"Yeah, get the jaws of life."

"You mean you want the door open."

"Yeah," the medic said, pissed. Moose doesn't look as bright as he is. "Don't you carry them in your rig?"

"You want the door open?"

Actually Moose was waiting for a "please."

"Jesus."

Moose grabbed the door handle, yanked the door off, and threw it into the gutter.

"What else?" he said.

I know I told that one before. If you were lucky enough to ride with me you might get to hear it several more times.

At my post, like most 911 crews, we ran 24 on, 48 off, 365 days a year. We got 8 hours straight sleep at night about as often as we ran all night without a break. We averaged five calls a day. At an hour or two per call, plus cleaning, restocking, posting in different locations, it was a full day. The most was a shift when I did 15 transports with 20 patient contacts—some "signed refusals" but also some double patient transports. You can carry two non-critical patients, or even two critical if back up is too far out to wait for. On average we got five hours a night, broken into at least two segments. We also napped during the day, and I was religious about getting home right after shift to make up sleep. No errands on the way. Drive home, big breakfast, omelet with bacon, capers and blue cheese, and sleep. Still, over time it wasn't enough. The sleep on shift, with one ear pointed at the radio, wasn't exactly real sleep, nor were day time naps. Running all night was doable; it meant a lot of good calls. I did 48 hours in a row once, taking a shift for someone after mine, and when I came back my wife asked me if I was OK. "Great," I said, "we did a full arrest and a gunshot to the head." Though the more experience I had, the more I came to appreciate BS calls.

Worst was a Fourth of July when we kept getting back to the station, and then being called out as soon as we hit the REM sleep. Ten minutes sleep every couple hours was far worse than none at all. I was starting to hallucinate sparkly lights on the white lines on the drive back to quarters. Plus you wouldn't believe the stupid things people do on the Fourth, and, worse, how they survive them with no more than boring scratches, bruises, and minor burns. Run cold water on them, by the way. Five or ten minutes. No salves. Not homemade, nor old wives', nor pharmacies'.

As for whether exhausted crews are safe drivers and attentive medics all the time, what do you think? Saves the taxpayer money.

When I was just starting, a more experienced medic advised, "Remember, it's not your emergency." It sounds cold, but what keeps you balanced, calm and focused is the sense that this catastrophe is your job, not your life

12 MCIS

MCI stands for Mass Casualty Incident. The phrase brings to mind 9/11, terrorist attacks, urban catastrophes, natural disasters, overturned busses full of screaming and bleeding passengers, but all it really means is that there are more patients than medics. A three vehicle collision with two crews available--four medics and five patients--is an MCI. More usually, a number of crews are available and a number of vehicles are involved.

The first thing to learn about MCIs is: locate all the patients. They have an exasperating propensity to be found wandering around, to go home and then come back, to be found in the wrong vehicle. Friends stop by and hop in the vehicle with injured people, injured people hop out for a stroll. Almost half of neck fractures are found ambulatory. So anyone in a high speed collision has to go on a backboard, strapped in with a cervical collar. For these with claustrophobia, or who have to sit up to breathe because of lung or heart problems, improvised solutions have to be found. (A KED, Kendrick Extrication Device, is a pain in the ass to put on, but it can immobilize a patient in a sitting up position.) People are thrown from wrecks and hide under bushes, unconscious.

You ask everyone in the vehicles to identify everyone who was on board, but they're not good at it. Especially DUIs. One drunk drove his vehicle off the road into the brush, where we found it, a beautiful new truck, almost intact, right side up with the roof crushed in. He swore his sister had been on board, he had talked to her after the wreck, and she might have had a head injury. Crew frantically searched the swampy woods. Fire flashlights examining every log. After a while, she walked up from her nearby house, where he had dropped her off earlier.

Any drunk with any kind of a head injury, no matter how small the bruise, has to be run emergent to a level one trauma center with neurosurgery capability. You get used to calling a jolly inebriate in to the triage physician as "probably just ETOH" (alcohol intoxication) but it's still "a head injury with altered mentation," even if only drunk, so only a scan can tell for sure if he's merely snockered or also bleeding intracranially. Drunks' brains will bleed from goose eggs which cause normal people only mild headaches.

We misplaced a corpse once. Drove the drunk driver to the level one trauma center, our back-up crew drove two passengers from the vehicle he plowed into to lesser hospitals with extremity fractures and back pain, and we heard at the hospital we had left a DOS behind. Dead on scene. The accident had occurred at night in heavy fog on a remote rural road. The drunk had swerved to try to avoid a pedestrian, whom he had seen too late, and who was unaccountably strolling remote from all habitation at 2 AM. The drunk had croqueted the victim into an overgrown roadside ditch, and then overcorrected his swerve to plow head on into vehicle two. Naturally he had reported none of this, the other vehicle's passengers had never even seen the pedestrian and there were no other witnesses. I'm not sure how the firemen even found the ex-pedestrian.

We took another call at a highway on ramp leading from a bank and insurance complex a few miles out of town on some beautiful landscaping with prime views of the surrounding pastoral scene. Normally we picked up anxiety attacks there, sometimes masquerading as chest pain. Amazing numbers of them. We joked that the banks' application form asked, "Do small problems seem insurmountable to you? Do you have trouble sleeping at night from worrying?" and only hired candidates who answered "yes." Though one time we took a signed refusal from an anxious chest pain who had changed his mind after his Xanax kicked in, only to find a security guard suffering a genuine MI.

This time, on the way there, we observed a pillar of black smoke rising straight into the air like Jehovah. We were hoping that wasn't our call.

It was. Three SUVs, all of the same make, model and color for some reason, had somehow collided as one or more pulled out of the complex's entrance onto the highway. The sandwiched one was burning lustily. We were anticipating having to fly burn victims to the BAMC burn unit, or not being able to get to them at all, but it turned out everyone had exited successfully. Various individuals from the bank were milling about among them.

We shipped two patients with another truck and took two ourselves. No one was seriously injured. It was all exacerbations of previous back problems, extremity fractures, neck pain and the like. We sorted them out.

After we got Cliff in the back with the sore back and the ankle fracture, a gentleman walked up and asked if he could ride along, as his wife was the lower back pain.

"Sure," I said cheerfully, "hop in."

We proceeded expeditiously but cautiously to University Hospital. I was making the turn onto Merton Minter, about a half mile out, when my passenger said,

"My neck hurts."

"Really," I said. I was sorting through an ominous suspicion when he said,

"Is it all right that my arm is tingling?"

"No," I said.

As I had feared, and as he now reported, under questioning, he had been in the SUV with his wife, had left to get something from the bank building, and had come back in time to join us. I considered pulling over, calling for backup, holding cervical spine until they arrived, and then extricating him onto a back board. We were however now at University Hospital.

"Hold completely still," I said. "Don't move." I called the hospital for some techs to assist us. They came out and helped Cliff unload his patients while I got a cervical collar. A couple techs brought a gurney around to the passenger door of the ambulance, and we extricated my passenger, fully immobilized, using a backboard, per protocol. I took him in, gave report and wrote it up. Fortunately, University is also a level one trauma center. I've never before or since extricated a patient from the passenger seat of my own ambulance.

Though, come to think of it, I did extricate myself once. We carry shears, mostly to cut clothes off injured patients, but also to cut bandages, and to amuse children by cutting through pennies. In theory, you can also use shears to cut someone out of a jammed seatbelt in a wreck, but I had never actually done this. Until one day I was sitting in the captain's chair behind a patient's head when I saw he needed suctioning. Suddenly compromised airway. I hit my seatbelt release. Hit it again. Shoved and yanked at it. Attempted to wriggle out underneath it. No luck. Patient now really needs suction. I yanked out my shears and extricated myself from my own seat.

Joe, head of Materials and Management, was furious. I asked him if he had ever succeeded in releasing the buckle. He pressed his lips together and looked the other way. The only thing I ever heard about it again was that I should have cut the female end. Remember that. Easier to fix and replace. I don't know why.

Usually, we found everyone, triaged them efficiently, backboarded them and lay them out in a neat row to be flown or otherwise transported out in priority of urgency, but plenty of times things don't work out as flawlessly as one might wish. These are accidents. And I don't just mean that the patents had failed to refrain from eating 24 hours before the collision, to be prepared for surgery; had neglected to urinate before the accident, to prevent bladder tears.

One of the first MCIs I ran involved three vehicles in a superhighway collision. We arrived on scene to find a sufficient number of first responders, and we soon had a backup crew on the way. Vehicle one had a driver and three passengers. The driver and rear passengers stated they were just fine and didn't need transport to a hospital. The front seat passenger, a 16 year old boy, hadn't had his seatbelt on, had smashed into the windshield, avulsed the skin on the side of his head so that you could see his ear through the flap of scalp, viewed from the top. He had experienced a loss of consciousness. He was presently alert and oriented, if freaked out, but clearly had a skull fracture. After triaging, I left my partner and some firemen to extricate him, back board, c collar, the works, and proceeded to vehicle two, undamaged. No one inside. There was however a gentleman ambling nearby clad only in boxer shorts, none too clean. He was the driver. He was perfectly fine, by his account, fully alert and oriented, stable vitals, no apparent distress, no visible or palpable injuries. I left the Basic EMT from the second crew, now arrived, to take a signed refusal from him. I told him to go do the same for the other three passengers of vehicle one. Why the gentleman was wandering around in boxers was an interesting question, but not one I had time to pursue at the present moment.

Vehicle three had a single passenger, the driver, who reported chest pain. Deformed steering wheel. Age over 55.

Two critical patients, two ambulances. I took the skull fracture, the other truck took the chest trauma. A fireman drove and we left a medic on scene to deal with the signed refusals. Everything seemed in good order.

But on the way to the hospital all hell broke loose. The other three passengers of vehicle one now said they were all injured, back pain, neck trauma, tender abdomens, what have you. Apparently, what they had meant earlier was that the 15 year old boy was the one I should take care of, and that they were OK only in the sense that they believed they weren't as seriously injured as he was. Two more ambulances were dispatched but, besides the time delay, I had left injured patients on scene, unattended except by firemen and one Basic. By protocol, you can only transfer care to medically trained personnel at your level or higher once contact has been established.

I survived professionally unscathed for three reasons. First, the other three really did have only minor injuries and the delay of care hadn't caused any problems. One reported his chief complaint at the hospital as "back board hurts." Back board pain is not an uncommon ER presentation, by the way. Second, critical patients can be transported immediately, and noncritical ones left on scene with first responders, if delay would jeopardize life or limb. Third, this was my first MCI, and while no one was truly happy with my disposal, it wasn't all that bad for a beginner.

We had a vehicle that had rolled over off a twisty little road, ending up on someone's front lawn, narrowly missing a tree. We found three patients. One had been ejected. He had a tender flank, possible kidney injury, another had neck pain, and a third a badly bruised knee, rule out fracture. Again, people who are seatbelted into modern vehicles survive horrendous crashes unscathed. These were kids and some of them had been less than scrupulous about belts and had the injuries to show for it. I loaded the kidney and the neck pain and gave the bruised knee to the Basic truck which backed me up. As we were loading, another ambulance screamed by. We found out later it was on the way to a nearby house to pick up another passenger from the wreck, who had walked home, and then his mom had called 911 to report possibly serious injuries.

We had finished loading, I was in back with the patients, when another boy walked up to Cliff, standing at the back of the ambulance.

"I don't remember the accident at all," he said.

"Why should you?" Cliff asked, focusing slowly.

"I was the driver."

The whole story was that he had an undiagnosed seizure disorder, had on this occasion seized while driving, and caused the wreck with five other kids on board. At the time, though, what we had was a patient with reported LOC post rollover (loss of consciousness).

I unloaded the neck pain, gave him to the Basic truck, loaded the LOC beside my kidney and proceeded post haste to the nearest level one trauma center.

So the first rule is, find all your patients. Triage. Get enough transport. Send the patients out in proper order. C-collar and backboard everyone. Stop any serious bleeding. Take vitals. Some of these things have to be done all at once. Hopefully, you have the hands to do this. If not, we have triage criteria for which patients are hopeless and must be abandoned in favor of ones who are salvageable, and for how to determine who is critical and who can wait.

En route is a busy time. You do a more thorough follow up exam, check interventions, start an IV, call in the patient report to the hospital, take a second set of vitals, bandage and splint if you have time, de rigueur if the bone fragments could cause arterial lacerations, all in an ambulance running at up to 90 mph. It's quite a sport. You feel very good about it if you've managed to do a lot of it well, prioritized intelligently, and given good reports both from the box and in the trauma room. Later, in order to practice what you might do better, you review the call, hopefully with other medics, and not in the middle of the night on your day off. Unfortunately, the service I worked for used the review process solely punitively, and so ineffectively that, like lightning, they struck the good and the wicked alike, insuring only that many uncertain newbies were handling a lot of calls, including the newbie investigators, who changed about every 6 months.

There's no such thing as a perfect run.

There are always things that could have been done better or more effectively or quicker. Something is always forgotten. If there are important lapses you kick yourself, again, hopefully, not for years.

If you're careful, work hard, study, are reasonably lucky, and have a talent for the job, you can expect to have many good calls and a minimum of bad ones. Those you have to live with, somehow.

13 NASTY GRANNY DAY; UNLAMENTED HUSBANDS

Calls tend to clump. One day you'll get nothing but chest pains. Another is seizures, or psych, or wrecks, or asthma. For a month you'll be hoppingly busy; another will be quiet. It's enough to make you superstitious.

We gave the days names, just as we named calls. The Kiss of the Spider call was the dude who walked into a local fire station for a spider bite. We have brown recluses and black widows but, after we got there, we couldn't find a mark on him. Here was a small speck that might have been a freckle. We offered to transport him, but he elected to watch and wait, after he calmed down. This was the same fire station where we picked up a 40 year old female EMT student who had become unresponsive during class. Even the experienced medics teaching the class bought it. She'd even managed to slow her heart rate down. I couldn't figure it out, since her vitals, blood sugar, muscle tone, skin color and cardiac rhythm were all normal for me, though she was still "unconscious." Until she woke up just enough, as we pulled into BAMC, to inform me that she had a deadly latex allergy. They still used latex gloves at BAMC. I told them everything. They were still working on it when I left. It was frustrating no one had any history on her.

She tried it again, and they decided to expel her from the class. She was not the first or last medic or EMT student I knew who generated symptoms to get herself transported via ambulance; just as there are firemen who start fires.

Nasty Granny Day started with a call at a small rural home where a 7 year old boy had slammed his fingers in the bathroom door. He had crushed the last joints of his middle and ring fingers irreparably. Mom, Auntie, and Granny were far more freaked out than our patient. Granny's first complaint was "you aren't EMS." That is, our private ambulance service, which handled Bexar County, within which San Antonio lies, is not the same as San Antonio Fire Department, which handles calls within the city limits. Our particular private service is the largest provider of emergency medical services in the world, handling, for example, the city of Chicago. By no means do its medics feel in any way inferior, except in pay, to SAFD. Quite the opposite. Because of our longer response and transport times, we carry more drugs and have more aggressive protocols than SAFD. But to Granny, they were EMS, and we were some kind of uniformed imposters driving a stolen truck.

There didn't seem to be any point in explaining any of this to her. She wasn't listening. Besides, we had our patient to take care of.

Then she felt we weren't reacting fast enough. I tried to calm her down, "I know this is an emergency to you," I began, intending to continue with an explanation about why we found it well within the bounds of things we could handle without strain or panic. That was the wrong opening. Not for the first or last time in my life, I chose the wrong words to express myself; not for the first or last time, I did not give enough thought to what was about to pass the barrier of my teeth. I have missed many perfect opportunities to shut up. She took me as saying that, while this was an emergency to her, we really didn't give a shit.

We packaged and bandaged him and set off. Cliff was in the back with the kid. He loves kids. I was in the front with

Granny. No love was lost between us. It was my prerogative to deny her transport, but it would have been stretching it, as he was a minor. Plus I didn't foresee what a perfect pain in the ass she was working up to be. I always figure I can get along with anyone for 15 minutes. We usually transported family members who wanted to go along, unless they seemed to be dangerous or out of control.

Which she was, actually.

Next, she somehow persuaded her brother, a police officer, to pull his unit up beside our moving ambulance, get me to roll down my window, and offer to "escort us" to Methodist Children's. I politely declined.

It was really one of the more bizarre offers I've received, far worse than the family members who, despite our explicit warnings, would on occasion follow our ambulance, running hot, with their flashers on, under the impression that they had suddenly become trained, experienced emergency vehicle operators, rather than idiots risking their own and others' lives.

In the first place, this officer wasn't protocoled to run hot through San Antonio, as we were. Second, I'm perfectly capable of running code all by myself. It's my job, in fact. Third, we're all explicitly taught that a second emergency vehicle should avoid running anywhere near the first. People see the first pass, assume all is clear, and then collide with the second. How he had escaped this basic bit of information in his own presumed training, I couldn't imagine.

Once he had been dissuaded from lighting us up, at the cost of not too much time, I still had her to deal with. We were running nonemergent, of course. True, the kid needed to go to the hospital. But his injury was not life threatening, nor even a threat to limb. Nor was a delay of ten minutes going to affect the progress of his treatment. For, while we always respond hot—you never know what you will find: it could be a distraught Mom who, obsessing about her daughter's cosmetic facial scratch, has neglected to mention that her bowels are hanging out of her abdomen (and, after all, a 911 truck is supposed to be an emergency response vehicle)—but we only transport hot under appropriate conditions. Ones that justify risking our own life and limb and those of everyone we meet en route. Not that, even then, we don't obey a lot carefully considered procedures to keep everyone as safe as possible. The rule is, we can disobey all traffic laws except school zones and train crossings. Otherwise the only criterion is "due regard" for safety. Of course, if you hit someone, it tends to be prima facie evidence of not exercising due regard.

Granny was continuously on her cell phone when she wasn't haranguing me. She kept up a running report to everyone she knew about her concerns, most of which focused on my many and varied incompetences. I very nearly stopped at a gas station to tell her she could either get out, or be removed by law enforcement, under arrest for interfering with an emergency crew. I decided to grit my teeth and bear it. 15 minutes not up yet.

"Now he's driving even slower," she wailed into her cell. And "have a hand surgeon meet us at the emergency room." I snorted internally. It would take an Act of Congress to get a hand surgeon to an ER for crushed fingernails. Perhaps one would go as courtesy for Queen Elizabeth. There's nothing a hand surgeon can do for a crushed last digit anyway, and, if there were, she would wait for the ER to page her after it had stabilized the wound.

Granny managed to get our patient upset. He was taking it all quite well before. So, unfortunately, as Cliff was bandaging the fingers, the kid yanked back, leaving the distal portion of his middle finger's last joint in Cliff's bandage. You can imagine how Granny took this. The digit was doomed anyway, was all this incident demonstrated, but I could see a suit in the offing. "Hey, I was just the driver." "It was like that when we found it."

What saved us was the multiplicity of the objects of her indignation. True, I had to write up an incident report, explaining why I had obeyed the traffic laws, but by the time good old officious Mack Cutter, Field Training Officer, was fully engaged in this congenial (to him) project, relieving me of the front line position, Granny had managed to get herself forcibly removed by law enforcement from Methodist Children's Hospital, who displayed considerably less patience than I had. My relatively minor incompetence faded into unimportance in comparison with the gross negligence displayed by the hospital. You have to prioritize. Concentrate your resources on the main front.

Not a couple hours later we took a call at a McMansion for diabetic complications. In the old days recalled by our textbooks, diabetic emergencies tended to mean undiagnosed or undertreated diabetics in sugar overload, with heavy, panting, Kussmaul breathing to vent acidity, sweating, malaise, ketoacidosis, hyperosmolar states or coma. In our practice, we saw some sick people with high blood sugars, but more usually we found insulin shock. Comatose or altered mental patients had either overdosed on insulin unwittingly, taken it without eating, or continued to take it even though they had thrown up every bite they'd eaten in two weeks. Some were just brittle.

We walked into an immense, beautifully appointed bedroom—shiny dark green drapes with everything color coordinated, it looked like an advertising spread from House and Garden, except less tasteful—to find a 20 year old, slender, pretty black woman bouncing on the bed, singing, and attempting to stuff bread down her mouth at the same time. The picture was instantly clear. She recognized low blood sugar, was attempting to ingest carbohydrates to fight it, and was not succeeding.

We took a D stick—a blood sugar. It was 23. Barely enough to sustain life. By the time Cliff had the sugar I had already started an IV. She was still bouncing, so this was an enjoyable challenge. A young person with good veins, so not that much of a challenge. No terror, just enough to keep our interest lively.

Then she collapsed back onto the luminescent green bedspread. Had she been white, her matte green skin would have clashed horribly. Being black, she just looked ashen. And, of course, clammy.

Cliff handed me the amp of D50—50% dextrose— and I squeezed the entire 25 grams into her AC vein.

Normally this is tremendously satisfying. You and five firemen struggle with a delirious patient to establish an intravenous line, you ease in the sugar, and the patient returns to normal within seconds. Another life saved. Everyone is happy. We've noticed the patients don't struggle as hard as they could. Perhaps they're too weak, or maybe some part of their brain is telling them we're on their side.

This time, however, nothing. Patient still comatose. Not good. D stick now 32. Not much better. I slung in another amp. I've never had to put two in a patient.

Still no progress. D stick still bad.

Our rapid exam was continuously in progress even as we were preparing for immediate transport, about to give up the "stay and play" mode for the "load and go." Cliff discovered an insulin pump attached to her waist.

I was for cutting the motherfucker the fuck off of her. It would serve it right. Basically, the pump was giving me the finger. It was daring me to slam more sugar into her, saying, in effect, "chuck in whatever you want, I'll just pump it right back out. I got more insulin than you have sugar. Make my day."

But Cliff, being diabetic himself, and also a wizard with technology, wanted to reprogram. (He took a brand new monitor we had never used or been adequately trained on into a full arrest, and not only ran it flawlessly, but managed to record all our interventions, drugs and what not, on the recording parameter designed for that purpose.) He was ready to call the number on the pump until I nixed. Too time consuming. So he managed to shut it off, not by cutting the catheter with EMT shears, but by pushing buttons and reading screens.

So another half amp gave us back our charming, bouncy patient, now calm and not singing. We got her a sandwich, as the D50 doesn't last, and took her to the hospital.

Where we met the interior decorator. Evil Granny number two. She was over 6 feet tall, at least in 4 inch spike heels, made up and dressed to kill. A terrifying spectacle, barely recognizable as human, surely not by expression. She could have walked into the academy awards and made everyone look insipid, or at least understated.

She was far too high in rank to talk to a medic, saving her overbearing charm for the MD, but she did ask me if I had checked her granddaughter's blood sugar. She didn't wait for my response. I was speechless anyway. Then she ordered me to get her granddaughter a warm blanket.

I actually did. Had it been for her, I would have discreetly disappeared. I had already transferred care to the MD, and I don't work for or in the hospital. But I had no beef against her daughter, and she could use a warm blanket. Besides, I like going in the heating cabinet and getting warm blankets. They're fluffy and warm. Patients love them. I love them.

Then I did disappear. I was beneath notice anyway, but this granny was, in my judgment, only marginally less dangerous than a suicide bomber. Let the MD take the hit. That's why he makes the big bucks. Which is another of the formulaic phrases we use, whenever we pass on something nasty to someone of higher rank.

Dang, now I can't remember Granny Three. I usually only remember patients for about 20 minutes anyway. People come up to me with shiny faces to thank me, and I have no idea who they are. They wink at me, failing to bring to my mind funny remarks I supposedly made. A friendly medic came up to me in a hospital and asked me if I remembered the full arrest I ran with him. I did not. "It was my first full arrest," he said. "I was a student." Still no bells. He was grinning at me. I looked at him. "You told me the patient died because I hadn't done the chest compressions right." He was laughing.

"No!" I said.

"Yeah, you did."

I guess you have to be a medic to understand. I was laughing myself by now, even though I still didn't remember the call. Of course he'd been doing compressions just fine, otherwise I would have corrected him. It just wasn't a viable patient. He'd realized that himself as soon as I winked at him. The shock and dismay wore off, and the ribbing had carried him through what can be a very traumatic experience for a beginner. They want it to be like on TV, where cardiac resuscitation works. You're all emotional and filled with adrenaline after the stress and exertion, pumping chest, and then you have a dead body under your hands. RX a little male bonding, which can work just as well for females.

"Yeah," he said. "You transported the patient as a courtesy to the family."

Well, that was my practice all right. After I was ready to pronounce, I would tell the family there was no hope, but I would be happy to transport if they would feel better. They might imagine the hospital could do something, 20 minutes too late, which I hadn't already done. They might feel bad if "everything hadn't been tried." Though of course it already had.

I preferred to leave the deceased in his home, without the alarums, expense and cold hospital light, but it wasn't my call.

The medic remembered my teaching with affection and gratitude, despite the rough handling. It goes to show that instead of sympathizing with someone facing a formidable obstacle, which may just further disempower him, sometimes it helps to throw another smaller, surmountable obstacle in his path, or jar him out of the funk.

So instead of Granny 3, let's segue onto "unlamented husband day."

For the first one, we responded hot practically the length of the county, the nearest available crew, shattering the night's peace with our flashing lights and screaming and wailing, to a strange rural home, far off on a country road. It was large, stone, rambling, full of dark, drafty, gritty corridors, huge stone kitchens, small rooms in cul de sacs, wandering over the field it occupied.

We had taken it easy en route because we were told it was "a probable." This meant someone had found a body she had judged to be unresuscitatable. These officers and firemen knew death when they saw it. They said "probable" DOS (dead on scene) because they're not supposed to pronounce except in really obvious cases. Still, no point endangering life and limb with high speeds.

The body was an obese, unkempt, smelly gentlemen in a back bedroom off a corridor not far from the huge ramshackle kitchen, but remote from the bedroom area where his wife had been. She told us he had gone in for a nap several hours ago, complaining he didn't feel well. He was flat line on the monitor, pupils fixed and dilated, dependent lividity under a massive pasty thigh, and even a touch of rigor in the jaw.

Usually people want to talk about it. Often they like to reminisce about the deceased. They show interest in the medicine or our interventions. She showed no interest at all. She avoided the men in boots tromping through her house. Relatives were showing up. She seemed a bit restless, but only because a number of the booted and uniformed rednecks browsing her house showed every inclination not only of sticking around but of summoning more personnel in the shape of medical examiners.

The house was dirty. That is, it was picked up, but had the air of some ancient castle whose inhabitants hadn't the resources to keep from falling into ruin. It was clear the husband had been distasteful to her even before he had created this mess.

There wasn't really any room for sympathy or empathy. She wasn't having any. Opaque. Just didn't feel like sharing her life with uninvited strangers.

We cleared and left. Maybe the officers or the ME discovered more of the story.

Many times I sat on the living room couch or at the kitchen table with a wife or children of a cardiac arrest, after the shouting captains had departed, leading a peaceful and soothing discussion of what had happened, who the patient was, what his personal and medical history had been, what we had done, why it had failed. The families of the ones we brought to a hospital, we saw only in the presence of physicians, or in passing the stretcher down the hallways of their home.

But even if survivors didn't want to talk, I'd still have to stay on scene until a police officer arrived. He would have to wait for the ME. Until the ME rules, the house of the deceased is a crime scene, and must be secured from evidence tampering. Once the officer was there, I could finish the paperwork in my truck if it seemed more appropriate, then give him a copy.

By the same token, an MD may interview the family and use his own judgment to DNR, or judge the case futile, but I must either see a DNR (Do Not Resuscitate) legal form or attempt resuscitation, no matter what the family says, or I think, would be the right choice. It would be worse than embarrassing if I took a wife's word for a victim's DNR wishes only to find later that she had offed him. Or wasn't the wife.

"Uh, well, this woman I thought was his wife said he didn't want to be resuscitated, and, uh, well, he looked pretty old and sick anyway....No, I don't know where she is now, but she said there were DNR papers somewhere...."

The second of the unlamented husbands didn't have a DNR either, but he was viable. Not really, but under the meaning of the act. He was in a back bedroom, on the floor on a rag carpet soaked in his bodily fluids, released by the loss of tone. His wife talked about a Do Not Resuscitate Order, but she could not produce it, so we were legally required to make all attempts to resuscitate him. What if she had been the cause of death?

He was in asystole, flatline, had been found down, unwitnessed, and so had a poor prognosis. I let a student attempt an intubation, and then I dropped the tube after he failed, which was quite gratifying, of course, One of the firemen pumping chest started gagging and had to leave to go outside and retch, much to the amusement of all. He'll never live it down. I think his nickname became "Chuck." But everyone in his station will have a ragging point of his own, of course.

We called it after our recorder said 30 minutes. "Man, doesn't time fly when you're having fun," I said. Everything had gone well, from our point of view, if not his. All the interventions had succeeded: the epinephrine, atropine and sodium bicarb infused into my patent IV at the right intervals and right dosages; strong, rapid chest compressions maintained throughout; intubation and ventilation through the endotracheal tube had successfully kept his oxygen saturation level high. But CO2 had remained low, indicating cellular respiration never came back. No sign of any rhythm on the monitor at any time.

Leaving my crew to clean up the mess, I walked into the living room, with my ubiquitous clipboard, to talk to the wife. No consolation necessary. Her sister was there and they were eager to discuss with each other and the sister's husband, "Where we go from here now that we can put our life back together." The deceased had been bipolar, apparently, and besides never drawing a happy breath himself, had made sure no one in his environment did either. If Poppa ain't happy, no one ain't happy. A member of my family met a similar description, but the wife did not want to hear about it. She wanted us out of there, the stiff out of her house, and her life reorganized into a semblance of decency and order, which had not been possible while the giant cockroach lived.

We cleared, leaving the sheriff's officer to wait for the ME. I wrote my voluminous run report, always multiple pages in a full arrest because of all the drugs, interventions and diagnostic work, and the high liability risk. The other crews, fire and EMS, were long since finished with the clean up by the time I was done and ready to hand a copy to the officer and the family.

Personally, I'd rather write a run form, no matter how complex, than scrub sticky gunk off a laryngoscope blade, using a horrible smelling disinfectant; reassemble and restock a drug box and jump bag; wipe down backboards and stretchers, and pick up and throw away bloody used garbage, but almost any other medic would rather do almost any other chore in preference to writing. That's why I earn the big bucks.

14 MORE SAVES

Lest this be getting depressing, giving everyone the idea that all EMS calls are fuckups, and that the medics, rather than being inspirational heroes, are perverts who find everyone's tragedies amusing, I should add a few more standard calls which are less memorable precisely because everything went according to Hoyle.

We go on scene looking at everything even before we see the patient. What kind of house? What does the interior look like? The neighborhood? Who's hanging around? What kind of yard? Cars, drugs? Tobacco? Alcohol? What are the first responders telling us about the patient or the background? What do they eat?

The second you see the patient you know a lot. Is he warm, pink and dry, or clammy? How's his breathing? Airway, breathing and circulation come first. Someone who is yelling "I can't breathe" is breathing just fine, though he may have other serious problems. Ditto anyone talking. If she's making sense, then her mental status, i.e. brain functions, thus blood circulation, are in some kind of order. We take vitals, a history, do trauma or medical exams, listen to lungs, feel tone. I MUST have my hands on the patient, though I've come to hate touching them without gloves. If I don't want to touch them at all, it means my instincts are telling me they're not patients, that is, not suffering any medical or traumatic crisis. Similarly, I hate sticking kids, but feel no reluctance at all if they need it.

Kids are terrified of needles. They'll suffer any amount of pain rather than receive pain killers, if the opiate requires a needle. A kid with a wrist bent into a fork shape, or a mashed humerus, focuses his fear on a tiny prick from a needle.

Depending on what we find, we either intervene or focus our exam toward our suspicions. We're pushing pushing pushing to get the medic in the back with the patient and the ambulance en route to the appropriate hospital. Or staying on scene to nebulize or inject drugs or work a full arrest. There are many variables, but they aren't infinite. The few that bamboozle you are treated symptomatically, and with diesel.

People who can't breathe are saved with nebulization, cardiac drugs, McGill forceps to remove foreign bodies. Asthmatic children, oldsters with chronic obstructive pulmonary disease or congestive heart failure, toddlers with objects stuck down their throats. Arterial bleeds are compressed or even tourniquetted. Broken necks are carefully extricated, cervical collared and backboarded. Lethally errant hearts are speeded up or slowed down with cardiac drugs or shocks. Many are saved, some are lost.

We arrive at a neat brick house to find a man pacing in the driveway. He's wheezing , choking and gasping, and despite all his efforts, his oxygen saturation is not good. We put him on 12 liters of pure oxygen via nebulizer mask. He improves markedly but only if he remains on O2 via continuous nebulization.

His story was that he was unemployed, visiting his ex-wife and her husband. He had asthma and was allergic to cats. Ex-wife had several (!). So he came outside but the asthma continued. He was still wheezy and constricted. We told him we had to transport him. He was reluctant. His plan was to wait till his wife came home with his medication and insurance documents. We told him he wouldn't survive if she didn't pull into the driveway approximately 10 minutes ago. He asked if we could leave an oxygen tank and possibly nebulizers.

This was a nonstarter for several reasons. First, we don't leave oxygen equipment. We don't even carry an extra regulator, so that would effectively deny us portable oxygen. An ambulance without portable oxygen is out of service. Then, we don't treat and leave generally. We treat if necessary and transport to definitive care.

He thought perhaps he could make it until his wife showed up. It was about 11 and she was due for lunch. I asked him if he planned to hold his breath for the next hour.

I called our on duty physician to see if he could add his authority to the persuasion. After we explained the situation, including symptoms and patient stats, the doc said, "He needs to be transported right now!" in an angry and exasperated voice. I told him he was preaching to the choir; the person who needed persuading was the patient.

I don't know what the doc said to him, but he agreed to be transported. This was going to cost him a lot of money he didn't have, but it was also going to save his life. Because, as bizarre and comical as his self-created situation might be (did his wife sue for custody of the cats? How did hubby No. 2 fit in?), there's no doubt that he would not have been able to hold his breath for an hour. There are people who say no one ever dies from asthma. They're wrong.

Asthmatics and other people with chronic lung conditions are given all kinds of potent at home medications these days. The problem this creates is that they may wait too long to call us. By the time their means are exhausted they are truly in extremis. Further, since the drugs they have at home are some of the same ones we carry, by the time we arrive we are down to only a few alternatives. We may have one or two more drugs to try and then it's a field intubation of a patient we have to paralyze first to get past his gag.

Another alternative we didn't have but some services were beginning to stock was CPAP: a mask attached to oxygen which provides Continuous Positive Air Pressure.

For example, we had a call for an 86 year old male with exacerbation of his chronic obstructive pulmonary disease—usually from smoking. His mentation was altered due to his inability, despite gasping for air at 40 breaths a minute, to keep his oxygen saturation above 86%: 95 and above being normal, and anything below 90, morbid. Further, he would soon be unable to maintain that kind of effort because he was becoming exhausted, and his muscles weren't receiving enough oxygen to continue to work effectively, nor his brain enough to command them. The technical term for this is "circling the drain," otherwise respiratory failure. He was a nice looking, white-blond, pink, hale and hearty guy, who was normally able to walk, talk and enjoy himself, despite a touch of Alzheimer's. We were out in the country, a minimum of 20 minutes from the nearest hospital, even running hot, and not counting securing him on the stretcher and loading.

He was, in other words, a candidate for chemically assisted intubation. This used to be called rapid sequence intubation, until someone noticed that there's not much about it that's very rapid, and haste makes waste. You get an intravenous line. You get your equipment ready and make sure everything is in order. You IV a sedative and then a paralytic. Some cynics say the only thing the sedative accomplishes is to make the patient unable to remember the ordeal. The patient becomes completely paralyzed, though still alert and conscious. Assuming he survives. Because, while normally paralyzing him makes him easier to ventilate via Bag Valve Mask, not always. That is, the next step is your partner applies a BVM to his face and begins to use it to breathe for him, as his breathing now stops. Then, after all of that proceeds according to plan, you lie him on his back, tip his head up, your partner puts a hand under his neck and lifts, uses his other hand to press down on the patient's cricoid in front of his neck, you slide a laryngoscope into his mouth, lift his tongue and jaw out of the way, visualize his vocal cords, and slide an endotracheal tube into his trachea, secure it, attach the BVM to the tube, and ventilate him via this equipment. If it all works. And, usually, it does.

And you don't do it just for fun, although it is a lot of fun. You do it when the alternative is letting him die. Because, all things being equal, if you have to be intubated, you want it done by an anesthesiologist in a fully equipped operating theatre, not on your living room floor by a kid in muddy fireman's boots, who may have never done it before. If you fail to be able to ventilate him, either via tube or bag valve mask, he dies.

A second reason to be reluctant to intubate is that an elderly patient with severe breathing problems must be weaned from the ventilator in the hospital rehab section afterwards. Not infrequently, this proves impossible, and the patient breathes on a vent for the rest of his unnatural life. Many people do not wish to live on a ventilator. I probably don't. They sign documents known as Do Not Resuscitate orders, which usually includes DNI, do not intubate. DNR/ DNI. It's quite difficult, legally, to remove someone from a vent. The patient is usually not mentally competent by that time to make the decision himself, legally.

So the first step is to find out what's wrong with the patient, in case there's a better solution. With a trauma history, it might be darting his chest to relieve the pressure of a pneumothorax: a punctured lung leaking air, which is then trapped between the lung and the chest wall, compressing the lung. This gentleman could be seen and heard to be wheezing and laboring to breathe. We knew it was COPD based on the history, but the wheezing and laboring exhalations had to be that, or asthma, both treated the same way, more or less. Had his lungs sounded wet rather than wheezy, and his breathing rapid, but without that effort to exhale typical of obstructive lung diseases, then we might have guessed congestive heart failure. Pneumonia would have been clearer lungs, less labor, localized crackles rather than burbly rhonchi, and a fever.

Then we had to decide whether to intubate, transport immediately or try something else. We were too far out to transport rapidly enough, given his bad shape.

I was saved from having to intubate by noticing that the patient had his own CPAP machine, which he used at night. He couldn't breathe well at night without Continuous Positive Air Pressure through a fitted mask. Family had tried it on him, but on the 6 liters of oxygen his oxygen converter supplied, it wasn't enough. Oxygen saturation still 86. Better than the 74 our nonrebreather oxygen mask produced, but not good enough. We, however, carry more powerful oxygen sources. The one thing an ambulance is never short of, nor shy about using, is oxygen.

Inexperienced nurses will sometimes berate us for putting a person with Chronic Obstructive Pulmonary Disease on too much oxygen, or leaving him on it when we find first responders have done so. These nurses know that COPDers can become dependent on supplementary oxygen. Worse, their brain's oxygen drive can short out over time, and they stop breathing. This is because, unlike normal people, their breathing has become dependent on the oxygen saturation drive: the back-up system to the CO2 drive which tells the rest us when to breathe. With the artificial O2 coming in, the O2 drive figures there's no need to take a breath. Unlike normal people, their brains have gotten so used to poor CO2 that they use the back-up system instead.

. But, "No, Honey," we tell the nurse. "That's your problem. For us, this run was a success. We took a guy in oxygen debt, heading for an untimely grave, and fixed it. What happens later is not an emergent problem." And that's what our textbooks reinforce.

When we attached this patient's machine to our oxygen tank, running at 12 liters, his SATs came up. He started looking out of his eyes again. I was also fortunate to find that my partner had experience with this equipment from working in hospitals. I asked if we could install the patient's CPAP in our truck. It had no battery, so had to be plugged in to work. We carry DC and AC outlets.

"Sure," my partner said.

So we gave the patient a few minutes on 12 liters to boost him to normal while we worked out our plan. He was in the front room of a little old farmhouse. Outside, after descending a homemade double step to ground level, was an obstacle course of gravel, pits in the lawn, old farm equipment and a discarded refrigerator. We lifted him onto our stretcher, secured him, and took him off his CPAP. My partner trotted out to the ambulance with the CPAP to attach it to juice and reset it. We stuck a nonrebreather mask on the patient at 15 liters. With luck, the firemen and I would be able to get him to the ambulance in five or six minutes. The nonrebreather should let him down slowly enough. I impressed upon them not to hurry. Even if it took too long to get to the CPAP, that was preferable to crashing into something or dumping the patient on his lawn. Besides looking really unprofessional, either would delay CPAP even longer. Act respectable.

With a strapping fireman on all four corners of the stretcher, this worked just fine. We were soon in route with a patient who was fixed. Good oxygen saturation, improved mental status. That is, he was still a bit demented, but that was a normal for him. En route I also nebulized vigorously—there's a way to do this through the CPAP.

This was an extremely successful call. But had the improvisation with the CPAP not worked, or had we failed to intubate, or intubated too late, I most likely would have lost my job. The questions asked would have been, why didn't I transport immediately? Why had intubation failed? Why had it taken so long? Why was I messing with equipment—the CPAP—which I had not been trained to use and which was not in our protocols, instead of transporting immediately? You almost never go wrong by rapid transport. They forgive poor skills, or failures to act, more readily than failure to transport. That's what ambulances do. Take patients to hospitals.

This patient might have survived the trip to the hospital without CPAP or intubation but not, in my opinion, without severe brain damage. An elderly, compromised patient with a poor medical history can't survive a half hour of oxygen SATs in the 70s or 80s. Intubation would have been the more standard alternative but, as explained above, it doesn't always work. Field intubations are not 100% successful. Bagging a paralyzed patient probably would have worked, but maybe not. Had the patient thrown up as a result of the ambulance ride, the paralytic, or the attempts to intubate, he would have aspirated his vomit, if we couldn't clear his airway quickly enough. He probably wouldn't have survived aspiration pneumonia. Intubated, he would have been vent dependent until, and if, he could be weaned.

Some ambulance services do carry CPAP. They report it drops their intubation rate by 80%. We did the right thing, but it required taking prudent risks, expertise of all kinds from different providers, a crew of people working well together, and some luck. An emergency call is always an improvisation but, like any improvisational art, the more you do it, the more licks you develop, and the oftener you practice equivalent situations.

We've had any number of kids with bad asthma attacks. Usually they respond to nebulization or subcutaneous epinephrine. We had a Viet Nam vet who liked epinephrine—it's basically speed—and, then, when high, loved his ambulance chauffeured visits to the VA even more, featuring multiple, gratifying chances to piss off VA staff, which was his preferred mode of socialization, being a lonely and alienating guy with PTSD. He had developed an uncanny ability to mimic the sounds and breathing pattern of severe asthma. Normally a faker holds his breath, or makes unconvincing wheezing sounds in his throat. You put your scope on his chest, and smile at him. You can hold the stethoscope there indefinitely. He can only hold his breath a minute or two. Then he has to take a nice deep one and you can hear everything in his lungs.

But this guy was able to fool both Keith, the medic after me on B shift, and me into immediately injecting him with epinephrine and transporting. He tended to become hostile, combative and abusive once he had his dose of amphetamines on board. I succeeded in keeping him calm, but he spat at Keith. You expect to get wet at my post, either sweat, blood, vomit, urine or wading through something outdoors, but this patient was also HIV and hepatitis positive, so Keith was less than pleased. I had found that if you let psych patients talk, and you listen sympathetically, subtly changing the subject when called for, they rarely give you problems you can't handle. Another medic I know—a very good medic—is 6' 6" and likes to use command and control, as advised by some textbooks. He got the shit kicked out of him twice.

Everyone needs a sympathetic listener. I would like one myself. Maybe I should call 911.

We also had a kid who had aspirated something. He was at a daycare. Cliff leapt out of the truck before it had stopped and I followed with the equipment, as per plan. He found a three year old with a provider bent over him applying an oxygen mask.

"Is that working?" Cliff asked.

"No," she said.

He grabbed the kid, flipped him over, pounded his back, and would have done some abdominal thrusts next, except the kid started breathing again. We listened carefully, looked down his throat cautiously—if he struggles or objects, this is better left undone as long as he's breathing—but we couldn't see anything or hear anything. The caretaker had no idea what if anything he had swallowed, but we bought her story because Cliff corroborated it. Otherwise "not breathing" can mean anything or nothing.

We transported. I watched carefully but the kid was in no apparent distress. Acting normal, breathing just fine, oxygen saturation at 100%.

As we walked into the children's ER a nurse ran up with a stethoscope. No sooner had she put it on his chest than he stopped breathing again. Whatever it was, had flipped back around or whatever and occluded his airway again. "I can't believe you're transporting a kid who's not breathing code two," she said (no lights, sirens or speed). We didn't have time to point out that if he hadn't been breathing we wouldn't have delivered a live patient to her.

She snatched the kid and a team worked on him in the trauma room. Two RNs, two techs and an MD. They couldn't see anything either, and whatever it was, was x ray transparent, so they couldn't see anything that way either. His oxygen saturation dropped alarmingly, but they managed to ventilate somehow, so not for long. Eventually they found a foreign object with a bronchoscope. So this remained a save, but it was near thing. Someone asked me later what I would have done had it happened in the ambulance. I had an answer, because that question had occurred to me too. "The same thing Cliff did," I said. "It worked once. Then I would've tried the Magill forceps." Which would not have worked, any more than they did in the ER. The next step would've been cutting a hole in his trachea and inserting an endotracheal tube. Had that not worked we would indeed have delivered a dead baby. You get lucky sometimes. And kids are remarkably resilient.

Army medics say, "You can always get an airway. It's blood you can't replace," trying to refute our airway, breathing, circulation (ABC) protocol. But not if the block is below the trachea.

What I learned from this is, if someone has an FBAO—foreign body airway obstruction—I want to see the foreign body. Or I want an alert, calm adult to tell me he's sure he swallowed it. He felt it go down. Otherwise I assume it's still in there.

You get lucky. I've never delivered a dead kid. I flew a couple who were near death out, but they became Airlife's problem. They were still alive when I handed them over. Waving goodbye. Poor little bears.

15 MISCELLANEOUS CALLS

Some of these I don't know whether to file under "saves" or "stupid pet tricks." Take the time Cliff and I walked into a suburban home, kind of unkempt lawn, not very good neighborhood, to find an "unresponsive " 26 year old female on a bed in the front bedroom. Her panicky sister told us she had no medical conditions, but she couldn't wake her.

We both had our hands on her instantly. Blood pressure OK, blood sugar OK, heart rate and rhythm OK, color and tone good, breathing good, oxygen SATs excellent, papillary responses normal. I'm checking her reflexes and Cliff is doing something to her toes to see if she responds to pain. Localizes pain? Withdraws? Abnormal flexion? Nothing?

Suddenly she leaps to her feet, yells, "Fuck this shit," and races out the door. We follow as fast as we can, but catch only a glimpse of her flying around the corner like a whippet.

We consider chasing her but by now we don't even know where she's gone. We elect to document the whole thing and clear the call. So, we resuscitated her, right? Or would you call this a stupid pet trick?

Like the 36 year old mother of three, also pregnant, who liked to frighten her kids to death by faking seizures. She had one in the ambulance too, supposedly. I gave her magnesium sulfate, which is what you give pregnant women who seize, but the picture looked all wrong to me. No incontinence, no post ictal period, she could answer questions while seizing, albeit in a weird voice, and her eyes rolled up when you pulled up her lids to check her pupils. I told her to save it for her kids. Some services allow medics to use some of their own judgment, but mine at the time insisted we do not diagnose, just follow the protocols. And it's true you can't tell for sure if someone is seizing or not, the brain being rather complex.

We see more fake seizures than real ones. An epileptic may seize during transport, or someone may suffer a rare and dangerous condition called status epilepticus, where they either seize again before fully recovering, or continue to seize, but generally a seizure is over by the time we get to a seizure call.

She's not the only mother who enjoyed terrifying her children in that way. We had another who "couldn't breathe." She convinced her panicked daughter, but not us, or the emergency room. "Why are you talking in that tiny voice?" the doctor said, his tone indicating she should knock it off.

We brought a couple of escape artists to South Central on the same day. The first was an elderly paranoid schizophrenic coming from the already described Sepulveda facility.

He behaved himself as long as I kept an eye on him. I outweighed him by 30 lbs., and, being paranoiac, he was unreasonably scared of me. I told the nurse about his proclivity for emancipating himself from restraints, but she said he'd be fine with just his arms tied down.

He did a kind of back flip and wriggled his way down the bed. He couldn't get any farther but, when I called her over to witness him in a half nelson off the foot of the bed, on the floor, she freaked. I helped her get him back up and better secured.

So when I brought the second elopement risk in, only an hour later, I expected she would listen to me this time. She said this patient would be fine too.

The patient wriggled her way loose and set off through the ER doors into the interior of the hospital. Normally, I would have called for assistance and impeded her escape, but this nurse had irked me. She came back to check on her patient to find her gone.

I was outside the cubicle door at the counter, working on my run form.

"Where is she?" the nurse cried.

"She went thataway," I said, indicating the depths of the hospital with my thumb. Nurse set off in hot pursuit. This being South Central, I imagine a Flying Dutchman or Wandering Jew type epic, with both of them, nurse and psycho, spotted from time to time, pursuer and pursued, in the Mobius corridors of myth. There have been enough times when nurses have handed me a frightening mess of one kind or another, with relief or even malicious satisfaction.

Elderly gentleman with cardiac symptoms.

"Do you have any cardiac history?"

"What?"

"Do you have any heart problems?"

"No.'

During my exam I discover he has a pacemaker.

"You have a pacemaker."

"Yeah."

"I thought you said you don't have any heart problems."

"I don't. It's working great. No problem."

16 LAST: BURNOUT

There are medics who can't handle stress, who yell at people on scene or who can't sleep at the station, but for the most part medics handle short term stress pretty well. If they can't, they tend not to choose this profession. Most medics in fact enjoy the adrenaline rush, are motivated to be Heroes who save lives, and will discuss really horrifying injuries or accidents with relish. They forget their patients 15 minutes after they deliver them to the hospital.

Long term stress is a different story. I had a colleague who did two tours in Iraq who described it very well. He said he lived in two different worlds. The first was the normal world most people live in with their friends, their families and their daily lives. The second was the stream of atrocities and horrors he witnessed in country. The problem, as he put it, was when the second world started to invade the first.

Partly it's the hours. 24 on, 48 off, 365 days a year, holidays, weekends, whatever. In 8 years I wasn't home on Thanksgiving, New Years and Christmas. Some years none of the above. I really didn't mind. I was neck deep in catastrophes, these shifts being holidays. But my family did. You do your best to keep up with sleep, you gobble spaghetti in the truck on the way to a call—angel hair, because it cooks in 3 minutes--but EMS engrosses everything. There's the studying beforehand and the reviewing afterwards.

It's engrossing, exciting. Enveloping. One of the things I liked so much about it, in fact, was similar to the reason my cat liked to go outside at night. During the day he's a cute fur ball dozing on a pillow, purring on someone's lap, moseying over to his food dish for a snack. But at night he's skulking through the underbrush trying to kill mice, or being stalked in turn by coyotes or bobcats. He might consider that to be real life. People who have served in wars, have tended to disaster victims in third world countries, have survived major illnesses or accidents, or seen their loved ones die: these are all of us eventually, but we quite rightly have sought to insulate ourselves as much as possible, and succeeded extremely well. But we harbor a sneaking suspicion that watching television or handling paper in an office lacks a certain authenticity, the kind we read about or watch, by preference, over the avant garde slice of life stuff their auteurs consider to reflect reality best.

It's like traveling by bicycle in an advanced country. Everyone else is insulated from weather and hardship but you're out in the elements. A few people in peaceful, prosperous, civilized countries are nevertheless out on the front lines. Soldiers, cops, firemen, certain medical personnel see firsthand the tragedies which most people see only on 3d rate news programs.

We don't like journalists, by the way, any more than predators like vultures. They'll betray a confidence or expose you, with malicious relish, for the sake of even a possible "story," and their only talent, besides an ability to wear makeup, is to speak clearly. They too tend to see themselves as experiencing real life, where at best they are only bystanders witnessing it.

It's empowering to be able to handle an emergency because you have the training and experience.

Conversely, EMS makes ordinary life seem unreal or unimportant. The hyperalertness and the observational skills you develop on scene can become eery when exercised on your front porch. As for example, when I arrived home late one night after taking a mandatory 12 hour overtime shift after my regular 24. I had my key in my front door lock when all the hair on the back of my neck stood up. As per custom, I instantly located what my Pavlovian reflexes were registering. It was my dog panting. I don't know what it is about the physiology of a dog, but an ordinary Lab doing his ordinary thing exhibits "symptoms" which in a human being would indicate respiratory failure. A human being normally can't take deep panting breaths at a rate of 36 a minute without passing out from hyperventilation. If he can, it's because he's working hard to maintain a precarious stability under threat from some morbid metabolic or cardiac or pulmonary condition.

Sam was of course perfectly fine. I stood down, as it were. Sleep deprived delusion.

A second cause of burnout, besides the hours and immersion, is what might loosely be called working conditions. The pay is poor. The hours are long. The conditions are problematic. Further, many of the calls can become just plain aggravating over the long term.

A major MVA with serious injuries remains exciting. I've had to dig a woman out of the ground she was crushed into, after we determined she was still breathing. An archeologist working with a neurologist would have done a better job, if they had several hours to work with, but we had none of the above. It was a drunk kid's mom. They had been coming back from a New Years' Eve party. He was fine, sitting, amazingly, still in the driver's seat, even though his roof had been sheared clean off. Mom had been thrown clear and rolled over. Fire had to support the upended truck, so it wouldn't fall back on us.

He asked about her from his ER bed. I said, "Well, she's still breathing." He started to cry, just leaking a little from the corners of his eyes. I doubt equally she made it.

This can be hard to take, but almost worse, in its own way, is the endless series of fenderbenders where no one is really injured, in all weathers and times of day, where you're getting signed refusals from all and sundry to protect the responding police officers from liability (why not? they protect us), or transporting 300 lb. people with back pain, anxiety, neck pain or bruises, on laboriously applied cervical collars and backboards (putting our backs at greater risk than theirs) to the nearest hospital, or to some distant hospital they prefer for one reason or other.

I've mentioned in previous chapters the calls we get from people who by no stretch of the imagination need ambulance transport. Another example would be a call we got at 2 AM. Climbing out of bed, we hustled, lights and sirens, to a suburban home where we found a married couple and a brother in law, all drunk and jolly, except for the wife. She was in the habit, she told us, of awaking at night to clean her ears with a Q tip. This time she had lost the cotton wad in her ear. In her impaired judgment, it could constitute a threat to her brain. What there was of it, at least. She was absolutely furious with her male relatives for laughing at her, and even more with us for not immediately extricating the cotton from her ear. We explained to her that not only didn't we have any such training but our tools, for example the Magill forceps we use to extricate foreign bodies from airways, wouldn't fit in the ear, even if we were inclined to exceed our protocols. We would be happy, of course, to take her to a hospital, which, generally, is what ambulances are for. "So," she wailed, "you're really no better than a taxi service." "Well," we said, "actually, we're considerably more expensive. You do get to lie down, though."

Sensing too late that this was likely to get me into trouble, I hastily added, "Now, if you were having a heart attack, we could possibly save your life."

The suggestion was made that she could possibly live until morning and then head to a medical clinic, if she had been unable to flush the cotton out with warm water by then, saving a lot of time and money in the ER. Not suggested by us though: we're told to transport everybody. I mean, what if she did have a heart attack? Or stabbed herself in the ear? We could be liable. We ended up taking a signed refusal, and she did call our main office. Couldn't sleep anyway, obsessing about the cotton in her ear. I had to write up an incident report. It was about the only time in 8 years when I had laughed at a patient. I regret it. It was unprofessional. I did turn down the beer they offered me, though.

"Assault" is another call which doesn't grow on you. You learn that assault means no one is hurt. If it's a stabbing, it's called a Stabbing; a fracture, a Fracture. A gunshot would be a GSW. Assault means someone got mad at someone and shoved her or punched her, without causing a "Head Injury."

Assaults always occur in the middle of the night. They always involve dysfunctional families all yelling at each other or officers or us, with drunken neighbors and relatives joining in so as not to miss any of the fun. It means bored police officers call you because they don't have the authority to clear a complainant medically, even if they know perfectly well she's not injured.

So Assaults mean you're staging around the corner for as much as an hour. You can't enter an Assault scene without police protection, for obvious reasons, but the police know as well as we do what's up, so they aren't in any hurry to respond.

At first these calls are very interesting. Broken glass, crying, yelling, a real show. It's no wonder the neighbors show up. But, pace Tolstoy, unhappy families are all alike. Over time, one Assault call becomes indistinguishable from the last. You come to realize these are not the kind of people you really enjoy spending a lot of time with. Eight year old kids yelling at Sheriff's Officers. People who really don't care what the neighbors think.

So, in time, up to three quarters of your practice becomes fairly boring. You might consider it pointless. It's dismaying to realize that, after years of seeing everything, you'd actually rather take these calls than true emergencies. I mean, really, who wouldn't? other than a crazy, gung ho new medic.

These considerations might lead you to want another job, but true burnout comes not from the BS calls, but from the bad calls. Long term stress. There's a limit to how many decapitations you want to see in your life, how many dead bodies you want to handle, how many tragedies and failures.

Every medic has calls that live with him. For most it's the dead babies. I had a few of them but, like Richard Hughes, I don't consider people to be fully human until they've got a few years on them, so for me it was the adolescent suicides. The poor little bears. A whole life in front of them, and they can't see they're not trapped forever, however bad it might be right now.

We found a 12 year old boy hanging in his closet.

We took a call at a decrepit trailer home listing into the weeds. Outside, an extremely suspicious looking man was pacing around. He'd called about his step daughter. We found her in fetal position next to her bed in a room the average adolescent would find unacceptably messy and dirty. She was cold as ice. Rigor had set in, so she was also stiff. She was wearing only tasseled panties. Her nipples were outlined in spangly silver paint which I was told was stripper regalia. She looked to be about 16.

We backed out and touched nothing, though we had momentarily picked up a scrawled note, mostly illegible, which seemed to say something about a boyfriend or love, and may have constituted, legally, a suicide note. After I pronounced death, this was a police matter.

That was far worse than the 6 month old we found still strapped to her car seat, which hadn't been secured to the seat, and had been ejected. After Airlife arrived and took over from me, she jerkily stretched out her right arm, as if waving goodbye. It's called decerebrate posturing, and means her brainstem is strangling as the swelling shoves it down into the spinal canal.

I'm going to tell the worst story now, though. I guess I've saved it for last. It comes with a warning. If you decide not to skip it, it may live with you, and wake you up at night for years, as it did me. That is, I don't have PTSD, I kept working, kept enjoying my life, for the most part nearly the same as before, but this boy lived with me. He has faded but not ever gone away. Fitzgerald observed that we are not one but many different people. It could be that one of the people I am, lost his will to live in a blue funk.

Oddly enough, it wasn't a call I took myself. If I had had the actual body to work on, it might have been different. Perhaps even worse, as it was for my partner, who did take the call. But having something to do with your hands, the action, the medical practice, probably would have given me a different handle on it.

It made the news for months, and lead to some changes in laws and procedures governing child abuse, though they were short lived. Investigators still turn over frequently and have unmanageable case loads. Modern society hasn't changed, and neither have political realities.

This was Christmas Morning. Cliff and the paramedic he was with, whose shift I later took over, walked into the disheveled interior of a brick home in a neighborhood which housed a number of bad actors, and a majority of perfectly decent families.

They found an 11 year old boy who looked, as my partner testified, like a death camp inmate. They guessed he was five, as he only weighed 38 lbs. His grandmother ran the household, as Elian's mom was in jail. She lived there with his aunt and three other kids who they treated reasonably well. This may seem odd, but the scapegoat has been documented since Biblical times.

Elian, though, she claimed in her trial, suffered "an eating disorder." It consisted of her starving him to death. Then she discovered he was sneaking up at night to raid the garbage can for food, so she duct taped him to his bed. After a while, he would cry, so she duct taped his mouth shut.

This is how his sister saw him, the last time anyone admitted to seeing him alive. She came into their room to get something. His last words were to her. He said, "I love you."

It makes you want to believe in angels and to understand why the most reverent observers have seen them as perverse beings.

The coup de gras, though, the cause of death, was blunt trauma to the head, though he would not have survived more than a few days anyway.

She and the aunt are in prison. Word on the street has it—we talk to a lot of felons and visit a lot of jails—that the other inmates know who she is and what's she's done and consider it to be their role in society to kick the shit out of her more or less daily. Felons have high moral standards. Very patriotic too. Sam. Johnson was right.

I'm glad they find it useful. It doesn't provide any closure for me.

I was getting pretty irritable with my family. Their problems seemed to be kind of trivial. They weren't dealing with them expeditiously. Sometimes they seemed to take on a kind of dreamlike pallor. I was thinking about something else.

I think I would have adjusted to the bad calls but not when you combine them with the low pay, long hours and the loss of interest in a majority of the calls.

I miss it, though. I'm glad I had the experience. It was not only the most interesting and rewarding job I've ever had, but it was my peak experience by some definitions. I thought everything was funny partly because I was exhilarated. "Manic" might be the medical term. Things like the patient we picked up because he was "chaking," per his mom. Spanish dialect for seizures--or just shaking. My partner, also Spanish and from an even worse background, was furious. "Chaking" he kept muttering. "Chaking. Can't even pronounce it. Ignorant pendejo. Taking him to the hospital in an ambulance for 'chaking.'"

Grand mal seizures are "oogly chaking." "He was chaking. It was oogly." Not to pick on Spanish people, blacks and white rednecks have their own dialect. Edema is "swole." As in "she's all swole." Smiley Might Jesus is spinal meningitis. Sick as hell anemia. Fireballs in the Eucharist: fibroids in the uterus.

My kids knew I "saved lives," but my daughter once asked me specifically if I had ever saved someone's life.

"Yes," I said. "That's my job.'

"Well, like, how many?"

"I don't know. Probably one a week." For five years.

They heard many of the stories at the dinner table. I taught my 11 year old son how to read all the cardiac rhythms at one point. It's a game paramedics enjoy. Not only fun but useful.

I'm not much of a believer, but I like to think I have a good end-times, last words story, equal to the many good answers that have been given to the question, "what would you say at the judgment seat?"

"What is the answer?" Gertrude Stein is supposed to have asked on her deathbed. "Well, what is the question?"

The atheist Heinrich Heine, asked what he would say if it all turned out to be true and he was summoned to judgment, said, "God will pardon me. That's his profession."

A professor told me he'd tell God, "I read your book." You may have to be a writer to appreciate that one. It's not an easy read.

I'm not by any sort of definition saintly. I probably don't even have a consistently good bedside manner, or enough sympathy and concern for my patients, let alone acquaintances, but I'll take a page from the story they taught me in grammar school (in the segregated, Bible belt South, believe it or not) about Abdul ben Bulbul. Not a Christian, thus.

"But," he told St Peter, "I did help my fellow man."

St Peter looked in his Book.

"And lo, Abdul Ben Bulbul's name led all the rest."

32813469R10081

Made in the USA
Charleston, SC
27 August 2014